Eat by Choice,
Not by Habit

Eat by Choice, Not by Habit

Practical Skills for Creating a
Healthy Relationship With
Your Body and Food

by Sylvia Haskvitz, M.A., R.D.

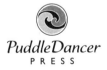

PuddleDancer
P R E S S

2240 Encinitas Blvd., Ste. D-911, Encinitas, CA 92024
email@PuddleDancer.com • www.PuddleDancer.com

For additional information:
Center for Nonviolent Communication
5600 San Francisco Rd., NE, Suite A, Albuquerque, NM 87109
Ph: 505-244-4041 • Fax: 505-247-0414 • Email: cnvc@cnvc.org • Website: www.cnvc.org

Eat by Choice, Not by Habit:
Practical Skills for Creating a Healthy Relationship
With Your Body and Food

PuddleDancer Press, Permissions Dept.
2240 Encinitas Blvd., Ste. D-911, Encinitas, CA 92024
Tel: 1-760-652-5754 Fax: 1-760-274-6400
www.NonviolentCommunication.com Email@PuddleDancer.com

Ordering Information
Please contact Independent Publishers Group, Tel: 312-337-0747;
Fax: 312-337-5985; Email: frontdesk@ipgbook.com or visit
www.IPGbook.com for other contact information and details
about ordering online

Author: Sylvia Haskvitz, M.A., R.D.
Manuscript Development: Jan Henrikson
Editor: Dan Shenk, CopyProof, ShenkCopyProof@aol.com
Index: Phyllis Linn, Indexpress
Cover and Interior Design: Lightbourne, Inc., www.lightbourne.com
Cover Photograph: © Big Cheese Photo / www.fotosearch.com

Manufactured in the United States of America

1st Printing, October, 2005

10 9 8 7 6 5 4 3

ISBN: 978-1-892005-20-5

Contents

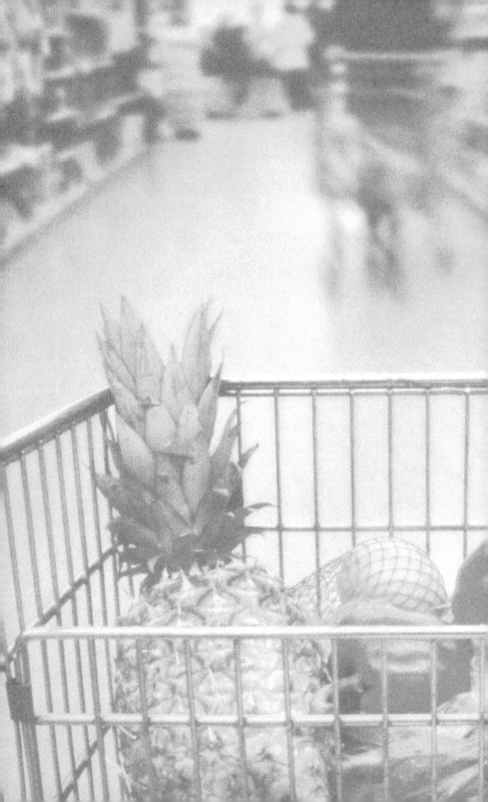

Acknowledgments

*"Gratitude is when memory is stored in
the heart and not in the mind."*

SAM N. HAMPTON

After writing and rewriting this book with deadlines, urgency, and passion, I've come to understand the meaning of acknowledgment and gratitude in a whole new way. I was always a bit surprised and confused when I read acknowledgments by an author of a book. How many people does it take to write a book anyway? I might as well ask: How many people are involved when we buy a loaf of bread? The farmers raise the wheat. The bakers bake the bread. The suppliers bring bread to the stores. The people at the grocery stores make it possible for us to have food. It sounds like a child's fairy tale, but it's true. It does take a village.

I want to celebrate my village—all the players who collaborated on this project with me. This process has been yet another reminder of how deeply connected we all are.

I would like to offer gratitude to Jan Henrikson, whose tireless hours of meeting, emailing, editing, rewriting, coaching, and encouraging made this whole project a meaningful delight. When I would spout hysteria about feeling overwhelmed or about my fears of having nothing to say, Jan would calm my inner critic and offer reassurance of the value of this project. Jan's connection to the topic and her fluency in Nonviolent Communication (NVC)™ were dream gifts in allowing this project to unfold in a precious, even delicious, way. Thanks also to her mother, Lois Henrikson, who generously provided her proofreading expertise and sadly passed away before the book was released, though not before the editing was done.

To Linda Prout, my friend, food buddy, and colleague, I was graced with your presence for a few days when you graciously offered to edit the first half of the book—especially "Sylvia's Soapbox." Linda's interest in and knowledge of anything related to nutrition fascinates and astounds me.

To my partner, Tim Lewis, deepest gratitude to you for enduring countless stirrings in the middle of the night while I raced to my office to capture my thoughts on paper before they escaped. I enjoyed your support of my work and your musings about your own experimentation with food and its impact. Thanks for always being a willing partner in taste-testing my latest concoctions.

To Mark Schultz, Katy Byrne, Elin Rydahl, Mary Mackenzie, Marie Miyashiro, and everyone else who shared their stories, asked questions, made comments, offered their support, friendship and excitement, I send waves of gratitude and acknowledgment.

To Marshall Rosenberg, Ph.D., founder of Nonviolent Communication, I am eternally grateful. You brought to life the consciousness and language I was searching for from age fifteen. To Kim Alison, my mentor and the one who I witnessed living the process in her everyday life, you were an inspiration for my own growth. I send special thanks to my dear friends, Bonnie Karlen, Lori Weinberg White, and Sedona Sunrise, who embody the meaning of friendship to me. And to my parents, Marvin and Dorothy Haskvitz, and sisters, Bonnie Belkin and Esther Haskvitz, from whom I developed my special connection with food and learned the role food plays in family, community, and health. If you were not named and know of your contributions to me, please include yourself in the acknowledgements with my gratitude.

Thank you!

Recipe for a Book:
How It Began

*"I am thrilled and deeply thankful to be playing
in my field of passion. I look forward to meeting
you in the field of compassion!"*

CATHY HARTMAN

As a registered dietitian and trainer in Compassionate/
Nonviolent Communication, I've been asked every
imaginable food and behavior-related question. Since I
couldn't answer every question in one book, I turned to
friends, neighbors, colleagues, the clerk at the grocery store,
and others for what they most wanted to know about
changing eating habits with compassion. What simpler way
to experience this process of discovery than through a series
of questions and responses—a dialogue—as Neill Gibson, a
consultant for PuddleDancer Press, suggested.

Jan Henrikson, a freelance writer, editor, creativity coach,
pet-sitter, and former NVC yearlong course participant, agreed
to play the role of interviewer. She asked the selected questions.
I answered spontaneously (for the most part). Two Basenjis and
a Rhodesian ridgeback quietly cheered us on, as the interview
took place at one of Jan's dog-sitting gigs. This was sheer joy
to me. Had Zera, my golden retriever and constant companion
of thirteen years, not died recently, she would have been
cheering us on, too. Maybe she sent me to these dogs instead!

While Jan transcribed the interview, adding generous helpings of rewording and editing, I ruminated during the night to bring her additions in the morning. We took turns stirring the words until we created something we hope you'll find flavorful and nourishing.

Now it's your turn. Focus on the questions that pique your curiosity, read them in order, or let the book fall open to just the right page. The point is: This is your journey now.

Bon appétit!

Introduction

"Face your stuff or stuff your face."
ANONYMOUS

Many of us are habitually at war with our bodies, treating them in ways we would not want to be treated or in ways we would never consider treating anyone else. We think we're meeting our needs by either satisfying our food cravings or bullying ourselves into denying them. In a dieting frenzy, we jump off and on the latest fad diets without ever stopping to discover what our real needs are. But we can feel something is missing. Chronically dissatisfied, we turn to the latest doctor, diet guru, tennis partner, or magazine article to tell us what to do.

My intent is that this book will help you uncover the missing link in your relationship with your body and food. This is not a diet regimen or prescription for instant results. I am not proposing to be yet another outside authority. Through the questions and answers in this book, I want to inspire you to access your own authority, your own power, and your own food and body wisdom.

These questions and answers offer an exploration of Nonviolent Communication (or Compassionate Communication)—and how it can guide you in your journey to make peace with your body. What are your needs? What are your feelings? Where are you focusing your attention in any given moment? Are you eating because your body is hungry? Because you want to distract yourself from boredom for a few minutes? Or do you want to meet other needs such as health, safety, security, love, nurturance, or protection? Or do you want to meet other needs, such as health, safety, security, love, nurturance, protection, or simply relieving a sense of distraction or boredom for a few minutes? The practice of Compassionate Communication can lead you to make conscious choices based on your needs rather than on habits that may not be serving you anymore.

"In the land of wine and brie, obesity is relatively rare," writes Mireille Guiliano in her book *French Women Don't Get Fat*. "We don't obsess about food, we're friends with it."

This is an invitation to stop focusing on food without thinking of much else ("obsessing") and start a new friendship. Not just for the moment, but each moment in a sustainable, even joyful way. Welcome.

Being Your Own Best Friend

"The one who stays by your side and finds a home in your heart is indeed a true friend."

ANONYMOUS

How can I befriend my body when it feels like a distant relative? I can't get rid of it, but I don't enjoy its company. And food is like an illicit lover. I'm always thinking about it, even when I don't want to. I don't even know what a healthy relationship between food and body is. What do you mean?

Imagine eating—or not eating—with a sense of harmony and balance because you're firmly connected to your feelings and needs. You know what choices to make in every moment. You eat in moderation, moving away from the table easily, without hassle, guilt, or the inclination to manipulate yourself into starvation. You savor six chocolate chip cookies straight from the oven on occasion without blame or shame. You step on a scale once in a while out of curiosity. You don't cringe and avoid the scale, and you're not wedded to weighing a certain number on the scale either. Instead, you're enjoying every sensual flavor of food—and of life, too.

❖ ❖ ❖

I need to diet, or I'll be out of control. Not being on a diet sounds scary and too good to be true. I can't eat chocolate chip cookies and lose weight.

Robert Fritz once said, "Diet is a path of feast resistance." Looking for a fight? Deprive yourself of all the flavors and textures you've come to love, and keep yourself in a perpetual state of hunger.

According to Fritz, the word *diet* is synonymous to many with starving yourself. You feel hungry because you are hungry. "There will always be a discrepancy between the actual amount of food your body is consuming and the amount of food your body wants. Solely counting and restricting calories to lose weight doesn't provide lasting results. But it's one surefire way to kick in your obsession about all the food you *shouldn't* be eating."

When you count calories and restrict your intake you will inevitably come to the place where you just can't stand measuring one more teaspoon of garlic sour cream mashed potatoes. Or you can't bear to watch your husband eat another bowl of peach ice cream, making "Mmmm ..." sounds with every spoonful. So you indulge. You not only eat the six gooey chocolate chip cookies, you eat the whole tray, the peach ice cream, and all the garlic mashed potatoes, and a bag of chips, too, for that satisfying crunch. That unleashes the dreaded *shoulds*. You should eat differently. You know better. Shape up. You should lose weight. "Look at me. I'm a fat pig. I can't even control myself." This outburst is followed quickly by "Screw you; I can eat what I want."

Now you're not only dieting, you've activated the demand/ resistance cycle, too. Demand change. Then resist it. As a bonus, moral judgment comes bounding in—you're "good" when you eat "right." You're "bad" when you give in. Moral judgments and compassion can't coexist. Without compassion, long-term change is impossible. According to Carl Jung, Swiss psychiatrist and author, "Condemnation does not liberate, it oppresses … We cannot change anything until we accept it."

Ultimately, you are having a relationship with struggle rather than deepening the relationship or connection with your body and your needs. Words like *should, shouldn't, can't,* and *won't* deny your own responsibility for the choices you make.

The process of Compassionate Communication has helped create peace between warring countries, rival gang members, hostile business partners, married couples, neighbors, and friends. Just imagine how tuning into your needs and feelings could help you create peace between you and your body, as well as the way you eat and the foods you choose.

Why are diets so popular if they hardly ever work? Everyone seems crazy about the low-fat, low-carb, or high-protein diets.

They do work—in the short run. We are a culture craving quick fixes. And fad diets are just that—fads, like hula hoops, hot pants, and disco. Here until the next diet sensation. They were never intended as permanent solutions. Instead, they provide the newest one-diet-plan-fits-all gimmick to hook you into ways to alter your body without acknowledging your unique life experiences, habits, choices, and physical makeup.

Say you go on the latest diet to lose weight for a wedding or a class reunion, or to get revenge on your ex-boyfriend. After the long-awaited event, if you haven't unearthed what needs and feelings motivated you to hold the weight in the first place, you'll likely boomerang back to your familiar eating patterns. Because fad diets are short-term and don't address your personal needs, you'll continue your yo-yo dieting, unaware of a different way of *being* with your body and food.

In addition, fad diets often produce health repercussions that may last longer than the diet ever did. When Oprah Winfrey launched her first highly publicized protein diet, I told my partner, "Mark my words, six months to a year from now she's going to be back up to the same weight and probably even higher." My prediction proved to be accurate. When people on high-protein diets regain weight, which is probable, they've changed their body's composition. They actually have a higher fat percentage and less muscle than before they began.

Years ago, when many of us chose low-fat diets, manufacturers responded with an explosion of low-fat products made tastier with added sugar. This strategy has unwittingly contributed to a host of such health challenges as osteoporosis, cancer, diabetes, and heart disease, not to mention tooth decay and obesity. Increased sugar consumption also has caused a surge of Type 2 diabetes in children. Once found only in adults, Type 2 diabetes is being diagnosed in children as young as *five* due to poor diet and insufficient exercise. Alarmingly, one in every three children born in 2000 will develop diabetes.

There is also the low-carb craze. Instead of fats, carbohydrates are singled out as the bad guy. We need carbohydrates. Whole-grain carbohydrates are an inexpensive energy source. They are the primary source of blood glucose, a major fuel for all the body's cells and virtually the only source of energy for the brain and red blood cells. Carbs also provide B vitamins that offer us stress relief and are vital to healthy hair, skin, and teeth. Note too, you can also find high quality carbohydrates in fruit, dairy, and vegetables.

Before clutching the next bagel, pause, breathe, and ask yourself: How am I feeling? What do I need? Follow this with a request of yourself. What choices are best for my individual health? What other needs am I trying to satisfy with any of these dieting strategies?

What makes you think people try to meet other needs by eating and dieting strategies?

Experience. In graduate school, whenever I was confused, frustrated, and overwhelmed while working on a paper, I would look for relief in the refrigerator. Or my house would get really clean. Or I'd surf all the TV channels. Back then, if I'd taken a moment to check in, I'd have heard, "I'm anxious. I want inspiration and creativity—now! I have no idea where to find it." I knew it wasn't in the refrigerator. But it was a way to distract and entertain me—a way to refrigerate my real needs.

A healthcare professional once said that he cherished his nightly ritual of snacking on cookies and milk while reading the newspaper. He more than cherished it. He couldn't do without it. It was sheer relaxation to him. After a few gentle questions, he revealed that his wife's depression medication also dampened her sexual desire. This left him lonely, longing for sexual and emotional intimacy with his beloved.

The moment he said that, something shifted. He suddenly saw his need for connection, saw the cookies and milk as edible substitutes. Now he has choices. He can open up to his wife or not. He can talk to his wife or keep eating the cookies. It's up to him.

Similarly, not long ago my partner's five-year-old granddaughter was so sad, she thought only one thing could help. "Do you have any chocolate?" she asked. I said: "Honey, you seem really upset. Do you want some loving? Would you like a hug?" "Yeah," she said, tears streaming down her face, forgetting all about the chocolate.

Instead of reaching for relief in a bar of chocolate, my partner, Tim, finds comfort in a disciplined diet, especially at times when his life seems out of control. Returning to structure soothes the anxiety welling inside. Never underestimate the unique, creative ways each of us has to satisfy the needs that call for our attention.

One way to discover the needs being met by your food choices is to list the foods you typically think of as *comfort foods*. When I asked my Eat by Choice food class to make such a list, they wrote: oatmeal, mashed potatoes, pudding, and pumpkin pie, all of which met needs for nurturance, love, and comfort. When I asked for a list of the foods people ate when they felt anxiety, they listed crunchy foods like Cheetos® and potato chips, meeting needs for relief and release. A woman noticed that crunchy foods were begging to be crunched to release the energy of anxiety. The foods were crunched into a soft, smooth texture. In that way, the actual chewing allowed the release and transformation of energy. Interestingly, the comfort foods were already soft and smooth.

When we grow conscious of the needs behind our food choices, we're also conscious of the abundance of choices or strategies we can use to fulfill those needs. Suddenly, the world is larger, and we expand, too. In one shift of awareness, cookies and milk transform from a need-hiding habit to an opportunity to make some far-reaching changes. Through one offer of a hug, the appeal of a sugary snack dissolves. The next few times you think about eating, tune in and ask, "Am I actually hungry?" You might be surprised by the answer.

As long as I recognize I'm an emotional eater, what's the harm in it? Sometimes I know I'm not hungry, and I eat anyway. I'm an emotional eater.

Awareness is the first step. If you say: "You know what? I want nurturing. And eating twenty-five potato chips is how I'm going to get it," at least you're aware that you're choosing the chips. Have you ever polished off a bag of chips unconsciously, not tasting a bite? You're left with nothing but greasy fingers, potato chip crumbs in your lap, and a vague salty sensation in your mouth. You're numb, but you still yearn for nurturing. You're stuffed and empty at the same time. You're more likely to reach for another bag of chips. As Anne Lamott says in her book *Traveling Mercies: Some Thoughts on Faith*, "I was a spy in the world of happy eating, always hungry, or stuffed, but never full."

All I have to do is be aware? That's it?

You don't have to do or be anything. NVC is about choice. Just as with the man with cookies and milk, when you're aware of your needs and what you're choosing this second, then options you'd never dreamed of before become alive to you. What do you want? Do you want a healthy lifestyle? Do you want to feel good and comfortable within? Then what choices are you willing to make every single day to make that happen? You can eat the chips, enjoying every salty crunch, you can call a loving friend, or you can curl up with a book.

How can I trust myself to make food choices that benefit me now? I've made so many food choices that I regret. What if I make more?

You're human. Chances are you'll make another regrettable choice or two in your lifetime. The difference is focus. This needs-based process of communicating internally focuses on being present and conscious with compassion—not being hyper-aware of every "flaw" and heckling or badgering yourself with insults. I like what Elin Rydahl, a practitioner of NVC says: "To give priority to oneself and one's own well-being without a sense of guilt or shame

> *"I have made a lot of mistakes falling in love—and regretted most of them—but never the potatoes that went with them."*
>
> NORA EPHRON,
> in her book *Heartburn*

is essential in order to reach the core of lasting change. If I can learn how to respect myself and my needs, can I also give myself the respect of a healthy body?"

If you make a choice you regret today—say, eating more pasta than you planned—Compassionate Communication invites you to say: "That was a choice I made. Thinking back about it, I'm regretful and wish I had chosen to tell my friend why I was upset instead of eating the pasta. I also know I'm human and am grateful to feel regret rather than blame. Tomorrow, I'm going to call her and attempt to resolve our differences. I really would like to make food and portion-size choices that meet my health needs." Then, instead of hounding yourself with your perceived misdeeds or inadequacies, let it go, knowing that you're in the process of discovering your needs moment by moment.

If you've made choices in the past that keep you up at nights, you could say: "You're no good. You'll never change. What makes you think this time will be different?"

Or you could cultivate the practice of self-acceptance: "At this point, I'm doing the best I can to honor my body. I care about my health and well-being and want to make different choices from the ones I made in the past. Looking back, I realize I've made choices in the past based on what I was going through in those moments. Sometimes I regret them because of the way they've impacted my body, health, and spirit. In this moment, however, I have compassion for me and for the reasons I made those choices.

❖ ❖ ❖

Real people don't talk like that.

This way of self-talk may sound like a mouthful, but as with any new language, it grows easier and feels more natural the more you speak it. The energy behind the words is more important than the exact wording. That energy of self-acceptance it embodies can be transforming.

Take a moment and ask yourself: "Where do I still need healing around the choices I've made? Are there things I regret? Do I want to give myself some acknowledgment for ways in which I wished I'd made different choices?"

Now empathize with yourself. For example, if you say, "Every time I came home from school upset, I ate a whole bag of jelly beans," you might ask yourself what need you were trying to meet. Were you lonely and seeking love? Did snacking on sugar meet that need for friends, fun, and understanding when your parents weren't at home to talk to about your day?

Let yourself grieve those times when you chose jelly beans over calling a friend or going outside and playing to meet your emotional needs. Now you're a conscious adult who knows that you can listen to your inner world at any moment for another satisfying way to experience love.

Reassure yourself: "I value health. In the past I've made choices to protect and nurture myself without considering the health implications as much as I would have liked. As a human being, I'm glad I'm feeling regretful and can mourn the decisions I've made without blaming myself or telling myself I should have behaved differently."

Blame is a battle cry that rouses your opposing inner forces. Blame is your judge, your critic … whatever pet name you have for it. It only feeds the demand/resistance cycle.

Acceptance and empathy open the pathway to powerful transformation.

This compassionate, empathic way of speaking allows you to stay connected to yourself at even the most fragile moments, moments when you would normally abandon yourself with judgment and shame and mindlessly eat the chips or ice cream.

Say you've put on weight in the past year, and your inner judge is running rampant. "I can't believe how much weight I've gained. Did I have no control over what I was doing? What excuse did I use not to go to the gym and work out?"

With compassion, bring the focus back to your feelings and needs. "I feel upset and frustrated and want reassurance that I'll make choices that are more in alignment with my health this year." Then tune in. Maybe you want some empathy for how hard it has been, with your hectic schedule, to go to the gym on a regular basis.

This self-empathy monologue is the antithesis to the inner critic. Gentleness with self also encourages change that lasts.

How will talking gently to myself help? How gentle can I be when I'm in the midst of intense food cravings? What if I have to have chocolate, and nothing else matters?

At the moment of real temptation, stop, even just for a second, and tune into your internal dialogue. Perhaps it's a whir of thoughts, such as this:

"I must have something sweet. I'm stressed out! Nothing will satisfy this craving but my favorite chocolate bar. Besides, chocolate relaxes me. But I've been telling everyone I'm on a diet, and eating chocolate doesn't fit into my diet. I'm getting my period, though. My hormones are out of whack. I need chocolate! I know Sylvia says we don't have physiological needs for chocolate, but I'm sure we must."

The first time you do this, you may find yourself biting into a chunk of chocolate before you've finished listening to the first thought. With practice, you'll be able to pause long enough to tune in to your needs and feelings and translate them into compassionate self-talk: "I'm torn! I'm sad and lonely and desperate for relief. There are lots of ways I can get relief. Chocolate is only one. Hiking with a friend might be fun. Maybe I'll open my art supplies and paint for twenty minutes. Which would I enjoy most in this moment, knowing that I also value health and well-being?"

Now, in this conscious state, whatever you decide is coming from a place of choice and presence. No *shoulds* about it. In these circumstances, if you choose chocolate, chances are you'll be able to truly savor a bite or two, whereas in the past even two chocolate bars may not have been "enough." You'll actually enjoy what you're eating without beating yourself up about it. That's because it's a gift you're giving yourself and receiving with peace. (Tip: My late friend Bernice Sachs said that when she ate quality chocolate, she was more readily satisfied with smaller portions.)

Is sugar addiction a part of what you're talking about? If so, how?

Sugar addiction is as much of a concern for some people as alcohol or drug addiction. You may not even realize how much sugar you're eating because it's found in all sorts of unexpected places and labeled under different names. Breakfast cereals, tomato sauces, and "healthy" mayo contain added sugars. Even a typical cup of fruit yogurt provides 70 percent of a day's worth of added sugar, according to the Center for Science in the Public Interest (CSPI).

If you're paying attention to sugar consumption, check labels for these ingredients: sucrose, high-fructose corn syrup, corn syrup, dextrose, glucose, fructose, maltose, turbinado, cane sugar, honey, and molasses. Sugar by any other name is still sugar. Though some "sugars" may wreak less havoc with your blood sugar and offer limited nutrients, you may want to limit your sugar intake if you're making a concerted effort to improve your health.

A chocolate lover for most of my life, I started noticing I was drawn to chocolate when I was upset, lonely, or irritated. Chocolate soothed, nurtured, and relaxed me. Since I enjoy experimenting, in July 2004, I decided to try an alkalizing eating plan based on the book, *The pH Miracle: Balance Your Diet, Reclaim Your Health* by Robert O. Young and Shelley Redford Young. Their premise is that all sugar is acidic, including sugars in fruit. By making your body more alkaline, you can cure disease and improve your heath status.

Although I craved chocolate for my first two weeks without it, the benefits of a sugar-free life have been astounding. I have no more urinary tract infections (UTIs). I used to get UTIs every few weeks. I'm excited because I often took antibiotics, which weaken the immune system and are hard on the body. Antibiotics can also lead to yeast overgrowth—candida, which contributes to sugar cravings. Now my energy level is higher than it has been in years. And I no longer crave sweets, something I used to eat daily. That's because sugar stimulates a desire for more sugar. (In the resources section toward the end, see tips on how to reduce sugar cravings.)

Today my diet is mostly vegetables, fish, nuts, whole grains, and an occasional piece of chicken or turkey. I satisfy any desire for something sweet with cacao nibs and cashews or slices of fruit and yogurt.

I'm not the only one who has romanced sugar. The average American consumes more than twenty teaspoons of added sugars per day, twice what the U.S. Department of Agriculture recommends. Annual sugar consumption has soared from 144 pounds per person in 1994 to 156 pounds in 2004. That's the weight of an entire person in sugar! In the book *Own Your Health: Choosing the Best from Alternative & Conventional Medicine*, Roanne Weisman, with Brian Berman, M.D., states that often when we crave something, it's not that we need it. We're actually allergic to it.

The spiking and plummeting of blood-sugar levels feed compulsive overeating. Mark Schultz, a recovering compulsive eater and NVC practitioner says: "With compulsive eating, I'd get short-term enjoyment and disconnect from my feelings. I'd feel some comfort, then get numb and feel depressed. I'd regret my behavior, condemn myself for it, then do it all over again." As his blood-sugar levels fell, so did his mood. He'd reach for more sugar to get the temporary high.

"It's easy to forget when you're feeling bad that what you need to do is stay with how you're feeling and figure out what you really need," adds Schultz. "It's a lot easier to just eat something, which is why addiction is so troublesome."

How can someone like Mark Schultz step out of the compulsive-eating cycle? Not by berating or depriving himself, but by something as simple and potent as the *pause*—pausing before eating your food of choice, or "holding the tension" as Becky Coleman, Ph.D., calls it. Coleman, a facilitator in food and body support groups, who weighed three hundred pounds—twice—has experienced firsthand how healing it is to develop the capacity to hold the tension that triggers a compulsive-eating binge.

In the midst of a craving, pause for five seconds to check in. How are you feeling? What do you need? What attracts you to the particular food you're craving? You can still eat your coveted food. But be aware. How does the first bite taste? What about the second bite? The fifteenth bite? Are you still enjoying the flavor? Are you making yourself eat it all? How does your body feel after the last bite?

NVC has helped many people get off the anger/rage cycle, to stop their anger from escalating into rage and possible violence by tuning into their feelings and needs. So it also can help you get off the compulsive-eating treadmill. Experiment. Find out what works for you. With continual awareness, increased compassion, and self-acceptance, you'll learn which foods and emotions trigger your compulsive-eating cycle.

As Schultz says: "At some point in this process, I realized I was slowly killing myself. Food became like my alcohol addiction. It was subtle, but it became a life-or-death thing. Now I experience myself just as I am. I experience my feelings. When I ate compulsively, I had no opportunity to do that."

He continues: "Abstaining from Krispy Kreme is part of a spiritual discipline like abstaining from alcohol. I identify deprivation as the feeling of craving with the assessment that

I'm missing out. When I pass a Krispy Kreme donut on a shelf, I feel the ache and remind myself what deeper needs I'm meeting by abstaining—specifically, health, self-respect, valuing life, hope, belonging in the world.

"My experience is that the ache leads me to recognize those deeper unmet needs. Although technically I might be 'missing out' on Krispy Kreme, I trust that I'm connecting with myself in a more profound, satisfying way. I trust that my desire for a donut will eventually subside as my desire for alcohol did."

What if I don't crave just sugar? Sometimes it seems like I'm addicted to all foods.

Meeting emotional needs with food at the expense of my body's needs may be considered violent. In another real-life account, here's how gentleness, compassion, and the pause, which are not sugar-specific healing tools, helped psychotherapist Katy Byrne release herself from her self proclaimed food obsession:

"I still cry when I talk about my eating disorder. I sometimes explode with grief for the years of suffering that I lived through, even though I've been free for fifteen years now. I rarely think about food anymore. I eat, or I don't eat. It's no big deal, but for so long I felt shame and chronic confusion. The longing for a normal life penetrated my pores, my cells. There was compulsion, thinking of food, wanting it to go away, hating myself, and trying things that didn't work. There was no time I didn't think about food: getting it, hiding it, swallowing it, being seen eating it. Food … was following me like a shadow nearly every moment.

"This morning I was overwhelmed with tears and a sort of shock. I had the feeling that a miracle had happened to me, that I had been walking through a dense, dark jungle for so many long, lonely years—and that now I can look back on it and feel free of that psychic drain, that constant obsession.

"Sure, I still watch the ten pounds come and go. I still go from a size eight to eleven, depending on my intimacy issues, sorrow, or anxiety. But I no longer live with the worry that food is my life, or that it will gobble me up. Now I'm concerned with pleasure, health, and looking to see what is going on with me emotionally. My body usually gives me a clue that I am stuffing something. It tells me what I need to look at and move through. It is my compass.

"I stopped putting myself in abusive relationships with food, people, places, or things when I started what I call my *hairball writing*. Getting my hairball out meant really seeing what was inside, viewing the real feelings coming out of my gut.

"I tried everything—twelve-step programs, diets, nutritionists, exercise, prayer—programs of every kind. The transformation came for me when I got my deepest hairball out. I found a little girl in me longing for love, who needed care and craved affection, and who thought there was love in the refrigerator.

"I remember the day I stood with the fridge door open and cried, staring at the food. I talked to my inner kid that day—before devouring the food. To that little girl inside me, I said: 'What do you really want? I won't beat you up anymore for it: just talk to me.'

"She said: 'I want food. Give me all that food in there. Get me chocolate-covered malt balls, wheat thins, donuts, and pizza.'

"I said: 'OK, I'll get them for you, but will that make you feel any better? What is it you really need?'

"She said: 'I really don't want to be bloated and sick. I want to be soothed. I want to be loved, and I want to feel full.'

"I said, 'What would that do for you?'

"That was the beginning of the change. I felt stupid standing at the fridge talking to myself. But that was the way for me: getting my hairball out."

Doesn't heredity play a big role in my ability to lose weight? You're forgetting something. Isn't there more to weight and eating than emotions and needs?

Heredity, hormones, or undiagnosed illnesses like celiac sprue (in which eating gluten sets off an autoimmune response damaging to the small intestine) may play some part in weight-loss difficulty. However, people also frequently use heredity as a reason why their bodies are not in alignment with their desired weight.

I think people may confuse heredity with lifestyle. David E. Schteingart, M.D., professor in the Department of Internal Medicine and director of the Obesity Rehabilitation Outpatient Program at the University of Michigan, says genetics are only 25 percent of your risk of being obese.

Cultural influences, personal lifestyle, and availability of food make up the other 75 percent. If you grow up in a household where fried foods, white bread, and sugary snacks are the norm, you may choose these foods as well. They feel like home. In that sense, you're inheriting certain tastes. However, those tastes aren't genetically imprinted. If you choose poor-quality fats and hydrogenated foods, you are actively clogging your arteries.

Or let's say your family members eat whenever they're upset. Until you become aware of this pattern or habit, you, too, may eat when you're upset without connecting to your needs. The choices you make at any moment impact your health.

If you choose to take your children to a fast-food restaurant six days a week, they will likely be obese and confront health concerns early in life. When one parent is labeled obese (according to standard height and weight charts) and the other parent is labeled normal weight based on the same charts, their child has a 60 percent chance of being obese. If both parents are obese, their child has an 80 percent chance of being obese (based on lifestyle choices). Here's it's worth reflecting again on the words of Carl Jung: "If there is anything we wish to change in the child, we should first examine it and see whether it is not something that could be better changed in ourselves."

In the last ten years, obesity has risen more than 50 percent. According to Dr. Richard H. Carmona, the US surgeon general, obesity is fast surpassing smoking as the number one cause of death from lifestyle choices. Three hundred thousand lives a year are lost to obesity. Its annual cost to society is approximately one hundred seventeen billion dollars. But these are just numbers. We can read this and say, "What a shame." What really motivates us to take action? Author Robert Fritz says it's not health threats from the world at large. It comes from inside, wanting something different for yourself. You may find inspiration in the most unlikely places.

For example, a friend of mine stopped eating hamburgers after watching the documentary, *Super Size Me*. In it, filmmaker Morgan Spurlock highlights the hazards of frequent fast-food eating and directly links it to the rise of obesity in the United States. According to Spurlock, in 1972 U.S. citizens spent three billion dollars a year on fast food, whereas today we spend more than one hundred ten billion dollars annually. He decided to demonstrate the hazards for himself by eating nothing but McDonald's food for breakfast, lunch, and dinner for thirty days. He made an agreement with himself before starting: If the clerk asked if he wanted his portion "supersized," he would say yes.

Doctors were shocked by how quickly there was a negative impact on this thirty-something man's health. His cholesterol shot up. His liver started to deteriorate. After fifteen days, his doctors strongly urged him to stop, citing health risks if he continued. Spurlock plowed on—against their advice and under the worried looks of his vegan chef girlfriend. He gained 5 percent of his body weight. Eventually, he felt good only after his sugar high from eating. That's how addicting the food became to his body. Imagine the impact on your child.

How do you get a child to eat more healthful foods? He's being bombarded by fast-food commercials, all his friends eat sugary snacks all day, and schools have soft drink and candy vending machines everywhere.

I'm gathering that you're frustrated and want some support in navigating your way around many of the "unhealthy" choices available to your child. In the same movie *Super Size Me,* Natural Ovens Bakery was highlighted for the impact of fresh, healthful foods on learning and behavior at Appleton Central Alternative High School in Wisconsin. There, so-called troubled teens showed amazing results when they changed their diets. Within one week of this diet change, teachers and administrators noticed students' attention spans had lengthened, and vandalism decreased. The school's most difficult problem was now a lack of parking spaces.

Natural Ovens Bakery did a five-year study at this alternative school with amazing results. Natural Ovens Bakery says if children continue to consume what they are now, they may be the first generation to die before their parents. That saddens me since we have choices about what we consume and what we give to our children. I not only want to preserve life, but quality of life as well.

How do we teach children to eat more healthfully? Short of force-feeding them through a tube in a hospital, you can't force your child to eat. Everyone has a need for autonomy. Kids want choice, and parents are worried about their kids' health. Parents often don't take their child's individual needs into account. They have to go to school, have to go to church, have to play with Floyd, have to, have to, have to.

Eating or not eating is one way children announce that they "*don't* have to." In fact, eating disorders often begin in children because that's the one area in their lives they have more control over.

This is understandably troubling to parents because they want their kids to eat all the nutrients they need to grow into healthy adults. Thus began the "Kids Are Starving in India Clean-Plate Club" threat and the "Try it so you'll know if you like it" plea. Instead of prompting eager eaters, this cajoling merely creates another demand/resistance cycle: "Nobody's going to tell me what to do. I don't have to. You can't make me!"

When we—children *or* adults—hear a demand, we naturally resist, even if it's the very thing we want. This stems from our strong need for autonomy, which begins at birth. At a nutrition lecture, Ellyn Satter, author of the book *How to Get Your Kid to Eat—But Not Too Much*, spoke about anorexic babies. When Mom or Dad demands the child nurse or take the bottle, the baby resists. The parents likely want to meet their needs to contribute to this new being, as well as worry about their level of mastery as new parents. The baby senses the urgency of the request, hears it as a demand, and resists, even though it may well be exactly what the child wants.

When I was a child, my father used to cook pancakes once or twice a year. If I didn't eat as many pancakes as he liked, he'd say, "Oh, you didn't like my pancakes." For him, food equaled love. If you don't eat all the pancakes, then you don't love me or value my contributions to you. Even as a child, I remember wanting my body's needs to be respected and my choices to be honored.

As an adult, when I visit my parents' house, my mother often sets food on the kitchen table while we're sitting around chatting: Reese's peanut butter cookies, pistachio cake, poppyseed cake, Hershey's syrup cake, foods I don't currently eat. "Eat! You're not eating enough," she'll say. That's a phrase that still rings in my ears from my childhood. In my younger years, I heard the message as a demand. I wanted choice and autonomy. Even when I was hungry, I'd say, "No, thanks."

Today, I often hear comments from parents like, "My kids won't eat anything but white or brown food" (macaroni and cheese, white bread, rice, chicken, and sweets). They're seen as "picky" eaters. For this very reason, Dr. Mehmet Oz, who was a regular on the Oprah Winfrey Show, calls them "the white kids" no matter what their skin color. Dr. Oz also said that you may want to continue to ask your children to try a new food—it may take ten requests before there is a willingness to check it out.

What can you say when you want to offer more variety to your child's diet? How about: "Can we explore different foods you like that also offer nutrition that will help you grow healthy?"

Or: "I know you enjoy sweet foods. Do you need something else, too? How about if we explore the needs you meet by eating cookies?"

Another possible overture—parent to child: "As a parent, I'm responsible to contribute to your life and to your health, so I'm making plenty of foods available that satisfy that need. I want to assure you that we'll find snacks and meals that are tasty and appealing to you as well. Would you be willing to try one new food a week to explore what you like?"

You may be saying: "Me? How can I say that to a kid who is screaming for Pop-Tarts? Or one who says, 'Stop talking!'"

Offer empathy: "Do you want your needs to be considered about what foods you enjoy?" or "Do you want a choice about what you'd like to eat without having to worry about your health?" Empathy invites dialogue.

I enjoyed a dialogue recently with Alina, the eight-year-old granddaughter of my partner, Tim. I grabbed the rice crackers from her lap when I saw her eating more of them than I was happy about. The following morning while cooking breakfast, Alina's seven-year-old sister, Anissa, found a spider web she wanted to disassemble. Alina shouted: "Don't! The spiders worked hard to make that web."

Anissa was focused on how spiders can hurt people. I suggested that spiders, like humans, probably hurt each other when they are scared. Then I told Alina that I regretted snatching the cracker box away from her without a dialogue. I told her I was concerned that she would develop habits of mindless eating that wouldn't serve her well in her life. Alina suggested that maybe I was also scared that cracker crumbs might destroy my computer. Empathy sure is contagious!

More important than the words you speak is the intent behind the words. You're providing appealing choices while setting boundaries. If you're concerned about what your child is eating at a friend's house, you can talk to the friend's parents or send over food that you consider fun and healthful. You're also teaching your children about food by your own choices, the way you speak about food, and your own level of self-acceptance around food.

Think about your own childhood messages—perhaps there's something about food that your mom, dad, grandparent, cousin, aunt, uncle, or friend said that you're still carrying around, being triggered by, and holding as truth. I agree with "Anonymous," who once said, "When you go home, of course your family is going to push your buttons; they're the ones who installed them."

I grew up with a girl whose mother padlocked the cabinets shut because she didn't want her children eating certain foods. What message did that send to her children? What did that say about which foods are acceptable and unacceptable? What dynamics do her children live with now as adults?

Are there any old messages you're still chewing on? If so, translate them into the possible feelings and needs of the person who said them.

How can I get his voice out of my head? My father always used to tell me I was too fat to eat chocolate.

This message is about Dad, not you. With Compassionate Communication skills, you can translate what was going on for your father. Was he scared? Did he want to protect you from pain he suffered while growing up? Did he feel sad about the food choices he made in the past or ones he still makes?

When a person speaks, his message is about his own needs. When you take the message personally, then you're locked into a few possible reactions, for example:

- You can feel lousy about yourself, agreeing with the other person's diagnosis of you.

- You can react defensively by attacking him.

- You can do both at the same time.

As you delve into the situation and see more clearly what may have prompted Dad's comment, you'll find yourself experiencing compassion for his fears. And you'll be able to acknowledge your own present reality.

You don't even have to talk with Dad to heal the situation with him. You can work through it on your own or with support from others. The key is to move through those stuck places that still influence you today by unraveling the feelings and needs of anyone involved.

You may discover lingering hurt feelings of your own that need healing. I'm guessing you may have felt sad and upset and would have liked understanding and acceptance, no matter what you weighed or looked like. I sense that you would have liked some compassion in that situation and feared you were being judged. Now you can choose to give yourself (that little girl) some compassion for her fears, as well as her desire to belong.

❖ ❖ ❖

How do I get past my childhood messages? My mom always said, "No dessert unless you eat all your fruits and vegetables." Now I see nutritious foods as a punishment.

Parents often use food as a way to reward their children for "behaving" or punish them when they're "misbehaving." For example:

- "If you don't scream while we're in the store, I'll take you to McDonald's for lunch."

- "Do that one more time, and no cake for you!"

One woman recalls being sent to bed without supper as a child as punishment. She lived in dire poverty and was starving much of the time anyway. Her hunger magnified everything: the voices of her family talking about how tasty the meal was, the sounds of silverware scraping plates, the scent of her favorite potatoes. That left a huge "food-print" on her. For years the sensation of hunger would panic her. As a result, if she was full, even overfull, she'd think, "I must have been a very good girl."

Another friend got Tootsie Rolls if she sat still for haircuts or stopped calling her sisters names. Today she rewards herself with food treats for every deed she deems "good." She's not the only one. Chances are you know some adults who say, "If I finish my project, I get to eat as much ice cream as I want." Or: "It's a special anniversary; let's treat ourselves to a gourmet restaurant."

In a system of justice based on punishments and rewards, we believe we deserve to suffer if we aren't following our diet. Some people reward themselves for dieting and for depriving themselves of their favorite foods for months by eating all of them in one sitting. Either extreme keeps us from being present to what we're feeling at this moment. Instead of viewing eating as a reward or punishment, ask: "What do I want to do regarding my eating, my body? What do I want my reasons to be for doing it?"

As for disentangling yourself from old messages about nutritious foods, did you hear the message "You should eat your fruits and vegetables" as a demand? Are you now resisting fruits and vegetables because you translated your mom's urgency as a demand? Are you eating out of habit rather than choice? Or are you still hoping to punish your mother—and needing empathy for the pain she stimulated in you?

Give yourself empathy for the pain you felt and may still feel. Feel the regret that you weren't able to hear your mother's message as her hopes and dreams for your health and well-being and instead interpreted her message as a punishment. Acknowledge to yourself the desire to enjoy foods that nourish you and keep you healthy.

You have a choice to look at what nutrients your body really needs. What fruits and vegetables can you get them from? You can look at blueberries and think: "Those are antioxidants. They eat up free radicals that can be causing disease in my body." (Free radicals are harmful chemicals found in the body that have been implicated in cancer and heart disease.) Do you want to fight against that? Or do you say: "I like blueberries anyway. Maybe I can add them to my yogurt today." Over time you'll see food as nurturing gifts that contribute to your life, rather than fighting against a voice from the past that's not helping you connect to your needs.

What if the voice I'm struggling with is my doctor's? My doctor says I have to lose weight, or I could be dead in two years. Where's the choice in that?

Let's translate that message with the Compassionate Communication process: "My doctor is concerned and wants to inspire change. Maybe he's worried about his ability as a doctor to help patients make changes to enhance their health."

Even though you may not have enjoyed or appreciated this doctor's delivery system, you want to check in with yourself to find your truth. Is there anything in what he's saying that really does make sense to you? Let's say your blood pressure is 140/95, you're five feet two, and you weigh 195 pounds. You could die of a stroke tomorrow. Does your weight concern you regarding your health and well-being? Or have you had enough of life? Are you ready to die, so the state of your health is OK with you? What's true for you? Do you want to live? Do you want to enjoy life? Do you have things to live for? If you choose life, you will choose strategies that meet those needs. If not, you will choose strategies to end your life.

Try on these responses:

- "I'm imagining a more peaceful life with more comfort within if my blood pressure lowered to 120/80 and my weight reached a place where I could walk up and down steps without being out of breath."

- "I want the freedom to eat what I want when I want, and I don't enjoy exercise. I will live with the consequences."

Next, ask yourself, "Do I want to make either of these choices no matter what anyone else wants?"

Other people's threats, warnings, teasing, and pleas typically don't catalyze powerful change. How many cigarette packages carry warnings from the surgeon general? How many people know about this threat and still smoke cigarettes?

More often than not, external advice activates a *should* reaction. "I should lose weight. My doctor says so." Or, "My partner (or husband or wife) wants me to lose weight."

This creates a push-pull between what someone else wants and what you want. You say, "What does that doctor know?" or "Screw you, if you don't accept me the way I am." You're filled with resistance because you think you have to, or should, or must. "You don't think I'm acceptable if I don't lose weight. I'll show you." From your anger and resentment, you make others pay for *"shoulding"* you.

You're likely living with an internal push/pull as well. You want health, and you want the freedom to eat what you want, when you want, in the quantities you want. When you *should* yourself, it's very unlikely you'll connect with your needs or get what you want. However, when you meet every moment with compassion, acceptance, and empathy, then you have nothing to fight against. You are your own ally. From that spaciousness, you are free to choose what you want and create a strategy in

which you are naturally satisfied. Ultimately, no food craving is
a match for compassion.

*Can you really change patterns you've had for more than
twenty years? Even if you discover your needs, work through
childhood food messages and get rid of your shoulds?*

Absolutely. "I was once again the world's oldest toddler," says
author Anne Lamott about learning to feed herself at age
thirty-three after years of bulimia. "I practiced, and all of a
sudden I was Helen Keller after she breaks the code for 'water,'
walking around touching things, learning their names. Only
in my case, I was discovering which foods I was hungry for,
and what it was like to eat them."

It's never too late or too early to begin again. Case in
point: When Oprah Winfrey interviewed Robert Downey Jr. on
her show, she asked him how hard it was to come clean after
years of drug abuse. He told her: "Once I decided to change,
doing something different was easy." The harrow-ing part was
clinging to a strategy that harmed him, all the while believing
that the strategy was saving him.

Play With Your Food

*"The discovery of a new dish does
more for human happiness than
the discovery of a new star."*
JEAN-ANTHELME BRILLAT-SAVARIN
(1755–1826)

Say you're ready to let go of a strategy that no longer works. You experience a sense of clarity that here, now, is the moment for change. You're ready to act on it. You feel it in your body all the way to your toes. What is one simple thing you can do right now to make the process easier? Enjoy. That's right, enjoy every gooey, crunchy, chewy, smooth bite you take. Revel in the pleasure. The more you savor, ever so slowly, what you're actually eating, the more satisfied you will be. The exquisite tastes—and infinite varieties—in foods constitute some of life's richest treasures and pleasures. Eating can be a sensual experience.

Imagine you're eating your favorite food right now. Is it salty? Sweet? Does the flavor burst in your mouth? Or does it roll slowly over your tongue? Is it cool or so hot that your eyes water? When do you enjoy eating it most? Where do you usually eat it? How did you first discover it?

I love whitefish salad on a bagel. The smooth texture, the sweetness of the tomato, the saltiness of the fish, the soft bagel with crunchy sesame seeds … all combine to create a true taste sensation. Whitefish reminds me of being a teenager, nurtured by my brother-in-law's parents for Sunday morning breakfast. Whitefish represents the best of being Jewish. It's food that nurtures and satisfies, food that is tasty and healthful.

Pay attention to the next bite you take. Sit quietly, without conversation or distraction. Give yourself fully to the experience. What do you notice? How do you feel while you're eating? Are you hungry? Does it crunch? Does it glide down your throat? Or does it feel like cardboard expanding as it settles? How does it feel in your stomach? What thoughts arise? Memories? Are you aware of any needs that are being met other than the obvious one of food?

I would love for people in our American culture to experience joy and satisfaction in eating. We're a society on the run, eating on the run. Some of us eat as if we were feeding quarters into an insatiable slot machine, one after the other, in restless agitation over that jackpot that never pays off.

The French, on the other hand, are known for savoring meals that last two or three hours as they commune with one another and the food. They eat croissants, butter, and cheeses, which are high in fat, yet they're thinner than we are as a whole. That's because they walk more than most Americans do. Their portions are smaller, too. They're eating higher-fat foods that satiate the appetite, needing to eat less to feel full. Our culture uses jumbo portion sizes to fill up the needs we're neglecting.

Think back. What is your activity of choice while eating? Do you eat in the car? Do you stand up at the kitchen counter? What does food taste like while you're eating and watching TV? How do your munchies taste when you're nervously working on a project? Now recall a time when you savored a meal. When you slow down, tastes and textures come alive on your tongue. You don't need massive quantities because you're actually receiving pleasure from each mouthful. Knowing you won't regret what you ate as soon as you finish heightens your enjoyment even more.

What does food taste like when you learn to balance your emotional and physical needs with your food choices? Is this something you would like to explore?

How do I get beyond the guilt to really enjoy food? Especially food I shouldn't be eating!

Let's translate the *should*. Is this a high-fat food that you're telling yourself is not good for you? Why are you saying you shouldn't have it? Reframe your thought process: "Maybe I want a smaller portion because it's something not necessarily as nourishing for my body as some other food choices. But I see how I can work that in if it's something I want." How does reframing that feel? What do you love that you eat in small portions?

Are you telling me I should enjoy eating more, and that would help? I don't really enjoy eating. I do it because I know I should.

There's that *should* word again! I'm guessing you don't enjoy food because some event or message from the past kept you from enjoying it. Did you always eat because you had to? Who did you see as putting pressure on you? What are some of your least favorite eating memories? What enjoyable eating moments do you recall? What made those stand out? Do you not enjoy eating because you are rushing to do things you would prefer doing, and eating takes time away from those activities?

Think of something you do enjoy, something you approach with a sense of lightness and play. Bring that sense of play and choice to food the next time you eat. Decorate your plate with color as you would when decorating your house. To spark more interest, eat only your favorite colors. Talk with your mouth full. There are no rules. No *shoulds*. Dress up. Dress down. Eat by candlelight. Make a picnic on the floor. Talk to your food. Pretend it's talking back.

Start noticing scents that you love, whether they're edible or not. Amber? Cinnamon? Vanilla? Rose? Pine? Curry? What kinds of textures please you? Silk? Corduroy? Liquid? Sand? Opening up to your senses in all areas will open up your food senses as well.

It's no wonder you have a push/pull relationship with food. Food elicits as many feelings as there are flavors—like excitement, joy, and safety. Our first moments in this world, we were fed milk from our mother's breast or from a bottle. Food also represents fear. We're bombarded by ads and diet books about what's good and what's bad for us. What's good this week is demonized next week. Woody Allen does a spoof on this in his movie *Sleeper.*

The owner of The Happy Carrot Health Food Store, Allen's character goes in for a routine operation and ends up cryogenically frozen. When he reawakens two hundred years in the future, scientists puzzle over the odd vegetable eating habits of the past. "Those are the charmed substances that some years ago were thought to contain life-preserving properties," says Dr. Aragon. "You mean there was no deep fat?" says Dr. Melik. "No steak or cream pies or … hot fudge. Incredible!"

Our ancestors might be just as incredulous about our modes of eating. For them, food was a means of survival. They embodied the adage "Eat to live." Many of us now "Live to eat" instead. Eating more quickly and chewing our food less not only diminishes our pleasure, it has our digestive systems asking us to make changes in our habits. More and more people suffer from the effects of digestive systems that are not functioning as they would like. More than sixty million Americans experience heartburn at least once a month. Fifteen million have it daily.

TV advertises a chemical solution. Love chili dogs, but your belly doesn't? Eat them anyway and take antacid. Instead of antacid, try taking a moment. Slow down, check in. What would make your eating experience fun now *and* a few hours from now? Are you not enjoying food because you're trying to find time to squeeze in a meal or snack and would prefer to be doing other things?

Are there any healthy foods that actually taste good? I love my food. But just about everything I eat is sugary and fatty.

As a child I used to pick a fresh tomato from our garden and eat it like an apple. The sweetness was delicious on a hot summer afternoon. Today it is more difficult to find tomatoes with flavor. Often produce is shipped to your local grocery store, which may take days. There it may sit on your grocer's shelves where repeated washing speeds up the aging process. Pesticides and genetically modified foods diminish natural flavors, too.

But flavor can be found. Just follow your nose. Take a whiff of the fruits and vegetables at the store. A ripe melon ready to be devoured will smell like melon. Tomatoes will smell like tomatoes. If they don't, they'll probably taste more like cardboard than the juicy fruit you long to bite into.

In addition to the grocery store, shop local organic farmers markets. If you are concerned about spending extra money buying organics, choose organic for the Dirty Dozen (the highest in pesticides): peaches, apples, sweet bell peppers, celery, nectarines, strawberries, cherries, lettuce, grapes, pears (imported), spinach, and potatoes. The lowest in pesticides are onions, avocado, sweet corn, pineapple (frozen), mango, sweet peas (frozen), asparagus, kiwi, bananas, cabbage, broccoli, and eggplant. Organic fruits and vegetables are often more flavorful and nutritious. Don't worry if they have blemishes on them. Conventionally grown food is kept blemish-free with chemicals your body would prefer you don't eat. If you're up for the adventure, grow your own fruits and vegetables. Do taste tests to see where you can find the most taste-pleasing produce.

If you are unable to buy organic use Sophie Uliano's Veggie Cleaner Spray. Combine the following ingredients and put in a spray bottle:
- 1 cup water
- 1 cup distilled white vinegar
- 1 tablespoon baking soda
- 20 drops grapefruit seed extract

Spray mixture on produce, let sit for 5–10 minutes, then rinse and enjoy.

The key to cooking tasty vegetables is buying quality vegetables and accenting them with condiments you enjoy, for example:

- Replace soy sauce with gomasio (a sesame seed and sea salt blend) or add olive oil and garlic to vegetables.

- Add tahini (a sesame paste) to your favorite vegetables or dressing.

- Try zaatar, (a mediterranean spice of sesame seeds, sumac, and thyme)

- Use organic, cold pressed, extra virgin olive oil. Add a small amount of olive oil to your salad with freshly squeezed lemon juice.

Cooking can be such a creative activity. Don't be afraid to alter any recipe to meet your needs. I am the "Queen of Alterations," taking after my grandmother, who everyone said could whip up delicious meals "in no time with no ingredients." In baking recipes I regularly cut the sugar and oil in half. No one misses those ingredients.

For a quick snack, instead of buying fruited yogurt, which is loaded with sugar, buy a full-fat plain yogurt with acidophilus. (It's more satisfying and satiating.) Add walnuts and cinnamon to it. Make it dessert-like for your kids; mix in a teaspoon of cocoa powder, carob powder, or poppy seeds.

Homemade hummus spread on rice crackers or used as a dip for carrots and other raw vegetables makes another satisfying snack. (Check *www.EatByChoice.com* for an easy hummus recipe.)

Watch your creativity come alive as you experiment. Feelings may come alive as well. Cooking may bring back childhood memories that enhance (or inhibit) your current exploration. Maybe the cook in your family told you to stay out of the kitchen. Or someone always corrected the way you cut an apple. As a result, you avoid the kitchen. When you do cook, you feel vulnerable regarding your cooking mastery and competency—and worry about sharing your creations.

If that's so, it's time to rethink and re-explore your feelings about cooking. Challenge yourself to have fun while creating something your body needs. As you do, you'll likely notice your tastes changing, too. Once-subtle flavors will blossom on your tongue. Since your tastes are more refined, foods will now seem naturally sweeter and saltier. As an added bonus, the less sugar you eat, the less you'll want.

I'm fascinated by the influence that cultural eating habits have on our taste buds. When I was in my twenties, I lived on a kibbutz in Israel and worked with two- to four-year-olds in the children's house. I loved to experiment with food even then. I'd offer the kids a piece of chocolate cake in one hand and a cucumber in the other.

Would you believe nine out of ten kids chose the cucumber?

Most Americans have built up such a tolerance for heavily sugared treats. But for those who are altering their eating patterns, flavors burst from unexpected sources. Our taste buds seem to cooperate with our intentions. Each time I go to Trader Joe's supermarket, I treat myself to a new taste sensation—one spice, snack, or meal I've never sampled before. This keeps shopping and eating an exciting, fluid adventure instead of a chore to meet a rigid diet plan. Shopping field trips with friends at local health-food stores is another way to avoid eating ruts. Sharing food choices can enliven any dining repertoire. Cook with your friends—experiment together. Alter recipes for greater health and well-being. Allow your creativity to go wild.

So what's wrong with eating unlimited vegetables? I have no trouble enjoying healthful food. More is better.

Again, the question is not about right or wrong but what need you want to meet. When people eat in quantities larger than the amount of food that commercial airplanes used to serve, they are likely eating more than their body needs. Can you get that need for nurturing, entertainment, and reassurance (or whatever need you've identified) met without eating a head of lettuce or a bag of carrots? That may work better for your budget as well.

According to author Robert Fritz, portion size plays a role in building health. In studies, mice that ate less food lived up to 40 percent longer. This fact begs the question: Are we killing ourselves by eating? Can we create better health if we eat less? The obvious answer to both questions is *yes.*

Is there a problem with "grazing" throughout the day? I like to eat small amounts frequently, and I'm hardly ever really hungry.

I don't see a major problem with that, although you probably want to give your body time to rest. Your body appreciates its insulin levels being stable. The digestive process taxes the body. If you're eating more than six times a day, you're not giving the body time to rest. If you want to eat more often than that, be sure you're adequately hydrated. Dehydration is often mistaken for hunger. When you urinate, if your urine is dark yellow, your body would like you to give it more water. If you're adequately hydrated, your urine output will be lemony yellow in color or perhaps lighter. Grazing also may occur because you aren't getting the protein and fat you need, so you aren't satiated.

If you drank a glass or two of water and ate three meals and two to three snacks, and you're still feeling hungry, you may want to check in with your emotional needs. You know the drill by now. What need is posing as hunger?

When is enough, enough?

Aside from our cultural penchant for eating large, sugar-laden portions, what keeps us from leaving the table when we're satisfied, not when we're ready to burst? It's hard to push yourself away from the table when you're just learning the difference between emotional and physical hunger. How can you tell when you're about to be full if you don't recognize when you're hungry? As you develop awareness of your needs and your sense of eating enjoyment, you'll also become attuned to your physical hunger cues. When one woman "feels empty" that means she's hungry. Other people experience gurgling stomachs. Begin noticing what hunger feels like for you. Note the sensations in your stomach, your hands, and your head. Where you do you feel your hunger pangs? Do you usually eat and eat and eat until you're suddenly bloated? Or can you sense when you're several bites away from satisfied?

Robert Fritz offers a Hunger/Satiation Rating Scale, which you can use as a guideline to practice hunger awareness.

   0. Beyond hungry—feeling weak or running on adrenaline.

1. Too hungry to care what you eat—you will tend to overeat.
2. Seriously hungry—you must eat now!
3. Moderately hungry—you could wait longer.
4. Slightly hungry—first thoughts of food.
5. Neutral—no hunger and no feelings of food in your stomach.
6. Satisfied—feel the food but don't feel full, no discomfort.
7. Slightly uncomfortable—a little too full, aware of food in stomach.
8. Uncomfortable—feel full, stomach distended.
9. Very full—want to lie down and digest.
10. Stuffed—so full it hurts.

From a physiological standpoint, it's best to eat when you're at "2" and stop when you're at "5." If you do this on a regular basis, you will become a normal weight. But there is nothing wrong with eating when you're at "3" and not stopping until you're at "6." Practice eating until you are no longer hungry instead of until you are full.

If you're looking for a cheat sheet to trigger inspiration, try this one adapted from Doris Wild Helmering and Dianne Hales' article "Think Thin, Be Thin" (downloadable from *www.Amazon.com*).

Physical hunger

- Builds gradually
- Strikes below the neck (growling stomach)

Emotional hunger

- Develops suddenly
- Strikes above the neck (i.e., a "taste" for ice cream)

• Occurs several hours after a meal	• Occurs at random times
• Goes away when full	• Persists despite eating
• Eating leads to a feeling of satisfaction	• Eating leads to guilt or shame

If you want, you can design your own hunger/satiation scale or cheat sheet incorporating your unique hunger cues. Remember, you're the authority. Only you can say when enough is enough.

Here are a couple of physiological nuggets that may help as you awaken your consciousness:

• Bob Greene, one of Oprah Winfrey's trainers, recommends not eating two hours before you go to bed. If you're feeling a little hungry, that means your body is using fat for fuel. When most of us feel slightly hungry, we want to fill up our stomachs, even though we're going to bed. We don't need nutrients then; we need to sleep.

• As I said before, our culture often mistakes thirst for hunger. When we drink soda, coffee, alcohol, or other sweetened beverages (including fruit juices), we are dehydrating our already dehydrated bodies. Sugar pulls water from our cells. Coffee is a diuretic. If you drink a glass of water and you are still physiologically hungry, eat something.

It isn't fair that some people can eat all they want! Some people never seem to get enough food. They can eat what they want and not gain weight. How is that fair?

My hunch is you're feeling envious and looking for some magical way to eat what you want while still meeting needs for beauty, health, and fitness.

Years ago I lived in San Francisco with my housemate, Kathleen, who struggled with her weight. She would devour fashion catalogs and say, "Oh, God, if I was your weight, this is what I'd wear." Her sense was "If only I get to a certain number on the scale, then I can choose these clothes to wear."

Well, I am at that number, and it doesn't have the same meaning for me. I'm forty-seven years old, five feet eight, and I've weighed between one hundred twenty and one hundred thirty-five pounds since I was fifteen. People have labeled me thin, slim, and other similar names. Although my weight has always been fairly stable, I've tried many diets and at different times imagined I was fat. My *what-ifs* are different from Kathleen's, too. Instead of wondering, "What if I could eat whatever I want and not gain weight?" I wonder, "What if I had five million dollars?" Instead of asking what-ifs, consider asking yourself, "What do I want?"

When people see me, they may think, "How can she eat that and stay thin?" Every moment, I make choices to maintain my weight and health. I've always been conscious of my food intake and the amount of exercise I do because I value health.

True, I may have been born with the nutrition gene. As a baby I'm told I refused to eat baby food from a jar. As a last resort, my mom bought a blender to blend whole vegetables and fruit. At sixteen I worked at Burger King. When a heavy couple returned to buy their second milkshakes, I said, "I'm sorry, were you just in here buying milkshakes?" When they responded yes, I said: "I can't get you another one. I'm worried about your health." I was fired later that evening, which was OK with me. I wasn't trying to be rude or flip. I did what I did with love and compassion.

I look the way I look because of the choices I make every day. That's true for 99 percent of the population. Some people have very high metabolisms. Others exercise so they can eat more than most. Most of the slender people you notice eating in quantities you consider large may only eat like that every month or two. You just happen to see them in their "large" eating moment.

Never mind them. What are your dreams for yourself? What do you value about your body? I know it's difficult not to compare yourself to other bodies when they're plastered all over magazines and movies. Although our society seems focused on "perfect" bodies, the media are showing people of all sizes more and more. In fact, there is a Dove advertising campaign for real beauty honoring every day people of every size. We've seen Oprah Winfrey in all her configurations—from medium weight to overweight to thinner. Many people in the media or in our families struggle, whether they're open about their struggles or not. And you always have a choice.

You can choose to celebrate your body. You don't "have to" wait for someone else to enjoy your body or tell you they like certain parts of your body.

Enjoy your own body. Move! Dance! Breathe …

My friend Bonnie was fascinated watching a particular woman at a process workshop on the Oregon Coast. Although the woman wasn't a classic beauty by society's standards and was considered homely by some, she freely whirled around the workshop, attracting more men than she knew what to do with. Her beauty shone from an inner sense of knowing and appreciation of her own value and worth.

What kind of relationship do you want to have with your body?

Are you saying I wouldn't be happier if I lost weight? I'm sure I would enjoy myself more.

Think about food as money in your checkbook. Each day you have a certain amount to spend. If you don't spend it all, you lose weight, and if you spend more than you have, you go into overdraft or gain weight. You pay a fee for going into your overdraft account. If you spend exactly what's in your checkbook, you maintain your weight.

Does that make you happier? Not necessarily. Money doesn't make people happy. An abundance of resources may meet needs for choice and ease—and may or may not stimulate feelings of happiness in any given moment.

Being lean doesn't automatically make people happier either. Some people relish the way they feel about themselves when their body is in alignment with their desire for health and fitness. Some people use weight for protection. What if they lost weight and still didn't find the "perfect" relationship or "perfect" job? That could be overwhelmingly scary. When the weight is gone, they're uneasy, exposed, and vulnerable until they explore their need for protection.

Do we *need* specific target numbers for our weight? No. We have *needs* for protection, health, well-being, vitality, and acceptance. Reaching a particular number on a scale is a *strategy* to meet needs and not a need itself. I don't need to weigh one hundred thirty pounds. I may choose to weigh one hundred thirty pounds because I know from experience that when I weigh one hundred thirty pounds, I enjoy the way my clothes fit (need for aesthetics). I enjoy the choices of clothing available to me (need for choice). I like the way I feel in my body at that weight (need for comfort). And I like the attention I receive from others. We contribute to our feelings of joy when we are satisfying our needs.

How important is exercise in this equation?

In 1990 I biked cross-country from the state of Washington to Maryland. For three months I rode seventy-five to a hundred miles a day, six days a week, pedaling a total of forty-five hundred miles. I may be a dietitian, but I enjoy using detective skills. To satisfy my curiosity, I did a pretest and posttest on my body fat and weight. My weight stayed the same, but my body fat percentage decreased four percentage points.

While I generally ate healthful foods, the quantities and combinations of foods I consumed amazed people. My leg muscles were defined like never before. My strength, endurance, and physical health were the best they'd ever been. My metabolism also has been higher as a result of this trip and seems to have stayed higher ever since.

Of course, you don't have to bike cross-country to reach a better level of fitness. Consistent exercise is powerful enough to boost your physical and emotional well-being in many different ways.

When you exercise, you'll likely eat fewer calories because moderate exercise actually curbs appetite. You may also experience an endorphin rush, which may meet some of the nurturing needs you met by eating when you weren't physiologically hungry. In addition, when you begin treating your body with compassion and care, you initiate a spiraling response. Just as violence begets violence, compassion and care beget compassion and care.

Exercise is key to your body being fit. Some experts would agree that being *fit* may be more important than being over-*fat* with regard to your overall health.

According to personal trainer Susan Tucker, the most important aspect of exercising is choosing a form you'll enjoy.

She also suggests ten to sixty minutes of aerobic exercise every day, depending on your level of fitness. If you're resuming exercise after a break, or just getting started, she recommends an initial ten to fifteen minutes. You'll want to combine aerobic exercise with resistance or strength training.

Aerobic exercise, or steady state exercise, is maintaining your target heart rate for twenty minutes. You may reach this state of continuous movement by walking, running, bicycling, or swimming. Resistance training is when you are new to working out with weights. As you build strength, your workout is called—no surprise—strength training. To develop an effective, injury-free routine, she highly recommends having a session or two with a fitness coach or hiring a certified personal trainer.

Zo Carroll, one such certified personal trainer suggests we look at exercise from both a physical and spiritual perspective—the mind/body connection. He says that when we move through exercise mindlessly, there is likely a "should" connected to the workout; a sense of mindless repetition without body awareness. To bring mindfulness to your exercise, feel and sense your body's reaction and changes as you work through the repetitions. Listen to what your body is telling you. Ask yourself if you're meeting needs for safety, fun, consistency, and pleasure. When you exercise, don't forget to include your kids and your dog. They also need to be active and fit—for their health.

Compassionate Eating: in Restaurants, on the Road

"One of the delights of life is eating with friends; second to that is talking about eating. And, for an unsurpassed double whammy, there is talking about eating while you are eating with friends."

LAURIE COLWIN
in her book *Home Cooking*

How do I avoid vending machines and fast-food places? It's easier for me to get into the rhythm of exercising and eating well at home, but I travel all the time. What's healthy on the road?

Plan ahead. Be prepared. Take along easily transportable foods: a sandwich; can of tuna or salmon; a mixture of raisins, almonds, and walnuts; an apple or dried mango slice. At a convenience store, grab a banana, bag of nuts, or cheese stick.

Avoid vending machines unless desperate. If that's your only option, then nuts may be your best bet. Granola-type bars are usually better choices than candy bars.

Before you leave home, search the Internet for health-food stores and restaurants in the areas you'll be traveling. Call the hotel where you'll be staying and ask for recommendations. Buy healthful snacks and to-go foods that don't require refrigeration. It might be fun to buy items you can't find in your hometown. If you travel to the same destinations regularly, keep track of their sources for healthful foods, just as you would tourist attractions or hotels.

When you eat out on the road, order a side of vegetables. Ask your server to split your entrée in two and box half of it before returning to your table. Dare to eat foods that aren't considered "breakfast" foods—enjoy the uneaten portion for breakfast or lunch the following day. Your body will be thrilled to get a jump start on the day by eating protein and vegetables.

Whatever you choose, don't wait to eat until you're starving. At that point, your serotonin level is so low it takes more food to reach fullness and satiation. You'll end up playing catch-up with food, eating more than you need in one sitting. That's why people who go without breakfast and lunch often come home and eat continuously from dinner until bedtime. Your body doesn't appreciate this—and neither does your mind. Studies of children who skip breakfast show they don't do as well in school because their brains aren't functioning the way they would with fuel and nourishment.

Does changing my eating patterns mean I can't eat out anymore? I love eating out, whether I'm traveling or at home.

I will translate the *can't* into a message of compassion first. Are you worried that making changes in your eating will not allow for the pleasure of eating in restaurants?

With food, as with life, options are always available. Servers are usually happy to accommodate their customers. Asking for what you want is just as important as connecting to your feelings and needs. In fact, it's the fourth step in the Compassionate Communication process: making a doable request.

As mostly a vegetarian since I was fifteen, I've had plenty of practice asking for what I want in restaurants all over the country. I may say: "I'm following a vegetarian diet and want clarity about a few items on your menu. Can you tell me if your soup is made with chicken stock?"

Or you may say: "I'm choosing to eat only certain foods, and I'm having difficulty finding what I want on your menu. Would you be willing to bring me a plate of vegetables as an entrée with sauce on the side?"

In this way you are responsible for choosing how much sauce you'd like to add to your meal rather than lamenting that the restaurant personnel are not in alignment with your nutritional needs and desires. As Marshall Rosenberg, founder of Nonviolent Communication, says, "When we blame others, we give up the power to change ourselves."

Your request can be as simple as asking the server in a Mexican restaurant to take the chips away. You may ask your partner, spouse, or friend to split an entrée with you and order an extra side salad or soup. You have more power to control your environment than you imagine. Just ask. Play with the notion of your needs as a gift to the person wanting to contribute to you.

What can I do during the holidays and at parties? It's the Thanksgiving/Christmas holiday season. I'm at a party. But I want to choose healthful foods.

Eat a snack before arriving at the party so you're not famished. Being overly hungry leads to choices we often regret.

Allow yourself the freedom to choose. Instead of restricting yourself, make agreements with yourself. Let yourself go through the buffet line one time and choose four dishes you'd like to try. Or talk to people away from the food table so you're not tempted to eat mindlessly. Drinking a glass of water after eating will fill you up and initiate a pause. If you're at a potluck and want to contribute, bring healthful food you love.

Limit your alcohol consumption. The ability to choose healthful food decreases with each drink. Alcohol also adds empty calories that don't contribute to your well-being.

Most important, check in with yourself throughout the party. Are you still hungry? Are you nervous because you don't enjoy social gatherings and you want relief? Are you hoping to find relief in the peanut bowl? Might you experience a sense of belonging in a glass of wine? Is your boyfriend flirting with someone? Are you anxious and seeking comfort? Knowing your needs and feelings in social situations helps you stay in alignment with your deepest desires.

Before arriving at the party—imagine your own success. Picture yourself chatting with someone and enjoying your conversation. Focus your attention on quality connections.

Supporting Others

"There is no downside for seeking to understand the essence of an issue or a person's point of view. It's amazing how much more creative and innovative people are when they feel heard and appreciated."

– DOC CHILDRE, developer of HeartMath

Supporting your spouse and choosing healthful foods at home—I've been married for ten years, and still don't know the difference between support and codependence.

Support is giving a gift that someone wants to receive— emotional nourishment in this case. You may choose to use Nonviolent (Compassionate) Communication to address your desire to offer support. The verbiage may look like this: "I've heard you say you want to make changes in your eating habits and food choices—and when I hear this, I feel happy and want to offer support. Can you tell me what I can do or say to give you support through this process?"

Codependence is worrying about someone else's decisions and their impact on your life. Codependence is being attached to the outcome or the strategy of the way you think things should be. It's different from interdependence. When you display codependent symptoms, it may be difficult for you to distinguish your needs from the needs of the other person.

You may be one person your loved one chooses to come

to for support. They may also enjoy joining a group for support. NVC practice groups happen all over the world. (Check *www.cnvc.org* for lists of possibilities.) Even though the topic may not be solely about weight issues, the practice you learn in these groups will offer the support you want for whatever changes you hope for.

How can you express your concern about your loved one's weight in a way they can hear?

First, you may want to get clear about what needs of yours are not being met, based on your loved one's weight. Are you concerned about health and want this person to be in your life for an extended time? Do you worry about their choices and how they will affect their own longevity? Are you less attracted to your partner than you would like to be?

Get clear about your own needs before approaching someone about their weight. When you have clarity, consider speaking with compassion about your concerns.

As author and speaker Marianne Williamson says, "Honesty without love is brutality." Expressing your truth with honesty in a way people can hear is a skill anyone can learn.

Say you're worried that your overweight spouse could have a heart attack tomorrow because of his or her eating habits. Pause. Tune in to your feelings and needs. Then speak from this place of consciousness. It may sound like this: "Honey, I'm afraid. Heart attacks happen instantly. You could die. Would you be willing to get a heart scan to see whether you have calcification?"

Or: "I care about you. I'm worried about losing you in my life. I want you to be around as long as you can be. Can you tell me how you feel hearing me say this?"

For me, weight is largely (no pun intended) about health issues, but for some, aesthetics might be a problem as well. If this is the case, you might say: "You know, you've gained about fifty pounds since we got married, and I'm not as attracted to you as I'd like to be. I long to feel excitement and connect with you in that way. Are you willing to consider making changes in your eating that we could both experience together?"

Refrain from such labeling, evaluative statements as "You're fat" and "You look like a blimp." I read a recent local newspaper story about a doctor who greeted a patient on the way into his office with the words "You're fat." I'm guessing the doctor was scared and needed reassurance that his patient would take care of herself.

Unfortunately, most of us are not motivated to change when we are called names.

When I was an adolescent, my father put a sign on my bedroom door that said "Garbage Dump." His need was likely for order. He was possibly frustrated that going into my room might have been a health hazard. Do you think I felt much like cleaning my room after that? It gave me permission to label myself a slob and act the part.

Labels create self-fulfilling prophecies.

When people box or label us, we tend to take their messages personally. Then our inner critic has a field day. It's unlikely we'll have compassion for ourselves or the ones speaking to us unless we've developed the skills to hear the feelings and needs behind the person's statement. How do you express what you want as a request rather than a demand?

Instead of berating your loved one every time they make a choice that doesn't support your requests or desires, check in again. Are you willing to allow your partner to choose what they want, based on their needs in any given moment? What are you willing to do to let go of the outcome?

How do I support a loved one in changing their eating habits?

First, determine what kind of support your loved one wants. You could ask: "I know you want to make some changes, and I'd like to offer you support. Can you tell me something I can do that would help you in this process?"

The person might respond, "I want you to keep your mouth shut when I'm making choices you don't approve of" or "When I'm making choices that you like, acknowledge that to me. Would you be willing to say, 'Wow, it looks like your clothes are fitting differently'?"

Here's another possible dialogue between two partners, both of whom are experienced with NVC:

He: "When I say, 'I really look fat today,' just acknowledge what I said rather than agreeing or disagreeing or adding comments. Say something like, 'Are you feeling depressed or upset thinking about how long it's going to take to reach the change you want?' Is this something that would work for you?"

She: "That doesn't work for me. When I hear you calling yourself names, I get triggered. I'd like more compassion around weight issues. Can you tell me how you feel when you hear me reveal that to you?"

He: "I feel touched by the caring you are expressing toward me. I want to be more accepting of myself. When you remind me of how hard I tend to be on myself, I am reminded to be more gentle, and I feel lighter about the whole situation."

What if my spouse isn't supportive? I've gained fifty pounds and want to lose weight, but my husband keeps making these huge meals and says, "Eat, eat." I think he likes plump women. I'm caught in a bind.

You're assuming that he wants you to remain at your present weight. Unless you ask, you don't know if that's true. You might say …

She: "I'm both pleased and frustrated when you make these meals. I like your food. I want to eat, and I also want to stay true to my own changes and choices. Can you tell me how you feel about what I'm telling you?" Or "I'm frustrated because I really want support. Is there something that's keeping you from wanting me to lose weight?"

He: "I'm scared because I like where you're at and, as much as you losing weight would be fun for me on some level, it also would bring up fears about other men being attracted to you."

She: "Are you worried and want reassurance that whatever weight I will be, I'll still have the desire to be with you?"

He: "Yes, I like our lives pretty much the way they are."

She: "I want to honor your fears and give you reassurance

that I will care about you, and I also want to honor my desire for health. Can you tell me how you feel when you hear me say this?"

He: "I feel happy knowing you want to take care of yourself, which will ultimately affect how long we'll be together."

Once you're connected with one another's needs, you may want to go to strategy.

She: "Would you be willing to keep ice cream, cookies, and soda pop out of the house?"

Instead of blaming your spouse for what they're not doing, you can ask for the support you truly want.

NOTE: Keep your environment one of peace and support in your efforts to make changes in your health. Instead of working on willpower, acknowledge foods that you have a tendency to eat more of than is necessary to meet your health needs. Keep them out of the house. If you want chocolate, for instance, and fear you won't be able to stop eating until the box is gone, go to a store that sells fine chocolate and buy a piece. Sit on the bench with your chocolate, and eat it slowly, savoring the creaminess or nutty crunch. Let the chocolate melt on your tongue and relish every moment of the experience.

What do I do when I see her eating her third piece of chocolate cake?

Take care of yourself when you see her making choices you don't like. If she asked you not to say anything, then she's very aware she's eating her third piece of chocolate cake. If it's upsetting you, you can talk to a friend or approach her directly. "When I see you make different choices than the ones you said you wanted to make, I'm confused and want clarification, and I also want to keep our agreement. Have you changed your mind, and have you decided you want to eat without restrictions?" Or, in other words: "I know I agreed not to say anything, but I'm having a hard time keeping that agreement. I see what's happening, and I'm worried about you. Before you eat the cake are you willing to tell me what's going on for you?"

Experiment with words that feel right to you. The heart of Compassionate Communication is connection—to yourself and to whomever you're speaking. Notice how it feels to speak and listen without *shoulds* and *musts*. You are not the food police to be avoided and rebelled against but an ally in this journey of transformation. NVC can greatly help you get in touch with your inside weather, getting clarity about what goes on in your inner world. It also can provide tools for listening to others with compassion. It can change your relationship with yourself and others, and you just might notice changes in your eating behaviors, too.

Sylvia's Soapbox

"Progress always involves risk;
you can't steal second base and
keep your foot on first."
FREDERICK WILCOX

Why a "soapbox" in this NVC book? As English philosopher and lawyer Francis Bacon once said, "Knowledge is power." I want you to have personal power to choose what works for you. By offering you additional information concerning food, nutrition, and well-being, I'm hoping awareness will lead you to choose in a way that best meets your needs. So here I am, up on my soapbox, a veggie burrito in one hand and my outrage in the other. I'm serving up my immediate passions and frustrations. With them come my desire for truthfulness, transparency, and a genuine concern for our health.

Trans fats belong in Transylvania!

Although the topic of nutrition is constantly explored, confusing and conflicting data and misinformation make understanding difficult. Many people throw up their hands in annoyance and irritation. What are you "supposed to" believe today after the umpteenth health update? Whom can you trust?

The US Food and Drug Administration (FDA)?

Can you trust the FDA to protect your health by approving only items that are beneficial to you? *O, The Oprah Magazine* (April 2005) states that members of the FDA have at one time or another been paid consultants at the pharmaceutical industries they are paid to be investigating.

In my twenty-plus years of rigorous food study and exploration, I, too, have questioned whose needs the food manufacturers and FDA are meeting when they fund studies. Is our health their main concern? Is it at least *one* of their concerns?

At a recent public forum on "Nutrition and Health: Food, Politics, and Society" sponsored by the University of Arizona Program in Integrative Medicine, I learned from a noted scientist at the Harvard School of Public Health that the USDA (US Department of Agriculture) is currently being run by someone whose degrees and papers are all related to animal health, not human health.

The more I learn, the more scared I become about what alleged protective agencies are allowing into our foods.

[NOTE: Beginning here in this section on trans fats—and continuing to the end of it—is **bold-faced** material from *Better Nutrition* magazine by Kimberly Lord Stewart, food journalist and author of *Eating Between The Lines: The Supermarket Shopper's Guide to the Truth Behind Food Labels*.]

Take hydrogenated fats, trans fats, and partially hydrogenated fats, for instance . . . These are the same names for fat molecules your body does not recognize and does not know what to do with! The body tries to use them in the same way as a liquid fat. When that's not successful,

the body stores the fat. The fat begins to accumulate and eventually leads to a whole host of problems, including Type 2 diabetes, arthritis, and cardiovascular disease. Trans fats lower good cholesterol.

In 1994, the Harvard School of Public Health estimated that at least thirty thousand people die each year of coronary heart disease as a result of eating hydrogenated fats. For each 2 percent increase in calories from trans fats, a woman's coronary risk escalates by 93 percent.

And yet, at the moment, **according to the FDA, trans fats, hydrogenated fats, or partially hydrogenated fats are found in nearly half of all cereals, 70 percent of cake mixes, 70 percent of chips and crackers, 80 percent of frozen breakfast baked goods, and 90 percent of all cookies.**

Dr. Richard Delany, M.D., cardiologist, internal medicine, and preventive medical specialist in Milton, Massachusetts, says there is probably no more important food issue than trans fats. Trans fats are worse for your health than butter, oil, or any other kind of fat.

What are trans fats anyway?

Trans fats are the fats that were hailed as healthier alternatives to the saturated fats we've been warned about since the 1980s. **Bombarding unsaturated liquid vegetable oils like soybean, canola, cottonseed, and corn oil with hydrogen gas and nickel or platinum makes partially hydrogenated fats.** Hydrogen atoms are inserted in no particular order. (Nature, on the other hand, does it in a very controlled way.)

When the incomplete hydrogenation process is stopped, unsaturated fatty acids are in varying stages of hydrogenation. Some molecules are mostly hydrogenated, while others are not. The double bonds have often shifted to unnatural positions. So many different compounds can be made during partial hydrogenation that it staggers the imagination. Scientists have barely scratched the surface of studying changes induced in fats and oils by partial hydrogenation.

The end result is that many of these altered substances are toxic to our systems.

Paul Stitt, M.S., owner of Natural Ovens Bakery and founder of the Nutrition for Optimal Health Association (NOHA), connects trans fats to the American obesity epidemic in a talk he presented for NOHA: "Americans eat more hydrogenated fat, more sugar, and more artificial sweeteners than any other people on earth—and experience more episodes of acute hunger each day than any other people on earth. Many people eat as often as eleven times a day.

Americans also consume less fiber than any other nation. Americans consume less omega-3, an essential fatty acid, than any other nation. And Americans do less physical work per day than any other nation. One of my greatest concerns in this moment is our use of hydrogenated fats." (NOTE: The author hasn't independently confirmed Stitt's claims.)

Dr. Barry Sears says it this way, "Today, for the first time in history, we have more overweight people on the face of the earth than malnourished people."

What was the FDA's response to this health hazard? In 2006 food manufacturers were required to label food products that contain trans fats. Some are doing so now. There is a loophole, however. Food manufacturers will be allowed to say that their product is trans-fat-free, even though that may not be entirely true. Read on.

I noticed this on a recent shopping trip. A particular margarine claimed it was trans fat free on the front label. But when I looked more carefully at the ingredients, I was disturbed to find partially hydrogenated fat listed near the top. I called the vice president of the company to clarify the discrepancy.

Without expressing feelings, and with judgments in my head, I blurted out: "How do you sleep at night? Trans fats are toxic to human beings. And you're willing to state there are no trans fats when they are clearly present? Help me understand the logic here."

She said that the FDA is OK with that verbiage if a product contains fewer than 0.5 grams of hydrogenated fats per serving. The FDA considers 0.5 grams to be a negligible health risk, though the Institute of Medicine says any level of trans fats is dangerous to health.

That means if you eat more than the single-serving size (which most Americans do) or eat a couple of trans-fat-free products at the same time, guess what? You're getting more than the 0.5 approved grams of trans fats.

What, I wonder, are the needs of the food manufacturers who create labels such as this? What are they appealing to? Clearly, they want us to enjoy the products they sell. They recognize that most of us live busy lives, so they want to make longer-lasting products for our ease and convenience. Hydrogenation meets both those needs. It increases the shelf life and flavor stability of foods containing these fats, as well as making food more crispy and flaky.

Wouldn't it be possible to meet these needs without jeopardizing the public's health? Can we find a win/win solution where we are not paying the price with our health and longevity? Scientific evidence shows that consumption of saturated fat, trans fat, and dietary cholesterol raises low-density lipoprotein (LDL), or "bad" cholesterol levels, which increases the risk of coronary heart disease (CHD).

According to the National Heart, Lung, and Blood Institute of the National Institutes of Health, more than twelve-and-a-half million Americans have CHD, and more than five hundred thousand die each year. As many of you know, that makes CHD one of the leading causes of death in the United States.

Do such food manufacturers consider my body and health needs? If not, it's up to me to make it a priority.

If you choose to rid your body of trans fats, the changes and benefits will show up in short order. You have the power with your lifestyle and the effects on your health.

Dr. Delany has seen blood triglyceride levels improve, insulin resistance disappear, and risk of heart attack and stroke decline when patients replace trans fats with healthful fats from flax, fish, oil, and nuts. He also advises women to avoid trans fats in order to lower their risk of developing breast cancer.

How? One step at a time. Start by replacing margarine with organic extra virgin cold pressed olive oil or grass fed butter. Eliminate trans fats and find such new sources of omega-3's as walnuts, flaxseed, and fish. Dr. Delany doesn't tell people not to eat any kind of fats, rather to find the right balance between omega-3 and omega-6 fatty acids. From processed foods people get a twenty to one ratio of omega-6 to omega-3 fats.

Surprising as it may sound, we do need fat in our diet, particularly those fats high in omega-3's. New research suggests that palm fruit oil and coconut oils, though saturated, are better for your health than hydrogenated oils. Other than breast milk, coconut oil is the only food source of lauric acid which has anti-viral and antifungal properties.

Fat is a major source of energy for the body and aids in the absorption of vitamins A, D, E, and K, as well as carotenoids. Both animal and plant-derived food products contain fat. When eaten in moderation, fat is important for proper growth, development, and maintenance of good health.

As a food ingredient, fat provides taste, consistency, and stability and helps you feel full. In addition, parents should be aware that fats are an especially important source of calories and nutrients for infants and toddlers (up to two years old), who have the highest energy needs per unit of body weight of any age group.

Have you noticed, as a culture, we keep eating lower and lower fat foods and our waist lines grow bigger and bigger and our health issues increase dramatically? It's not so much about the amount of fat, but the kind of fat we're eating. I know, I know, you remember the 60's–80's when vegetable fat was touted as healthy. It was a scam! Heart disease has gone rampant since vegetable oils have been used. Don't take my word for it. Check out the latest reseach at *www.westonaprice.org*.

Fats I would recommend: grass fed butter (Kerrygold, for example at Trader Joe's), ghee, sesame oil, coconut oil, olive oil, flax seed oil, fish oil, lard, chicken, goose, and duck fat.

It's your body. It's your choice. Read the labels. Know what you're feeding your precious body—that you were given *only one of* in this lifetime. Don't allow food manufacturers to meet their needs at your health's expense!

Eating instead of grieving

While I worked as a dietitian in an eating disorders program in a Minneapolis hospital, the staff noticed something curious. In our own informal study, we realized that a large portion of our client load had experienced the death of a sibling in childhood.

> *"Ain't that just the way life is? No time for grieving."*
>
> Sierra Tucson Treatment Center participant

Is disordered eating just another outcome of not grieving?

At the University of Arizona in early preseason basketball, on the second day of practice, a new recruit keeled over and died of heatstroke. He was just eighteen.

Practice was canceled the next day in honor of this young freshman. The following day, less than twenty-four hours after this teenager's death, the radio announcer stated, "The team is *finally* getting back to normal."

In Judaism, Shiva (seven days of sitting with mourners in their home) has often been shortened to three or four days due to people's busy schedules.

Celebrations occur with festive eats. Mourning, on the other hand, seems to be pushed underground for fear of experiencing unpleasant feelings, sometimes in the guise of protecting people from pain.

Is the use and abuse of food often related to our lack of mourning, grieving, and acknowledging our pain? Or as Gabriel Cousens says: "There's never enough food to feed a hungry soul."

Are we a culture afraid to feel our feelings? Are we protecting ourselves for fear if we open the floodgates, the tears may never stop? Do we then stuff our faces, drink ourselves into oblivion, and drug ourselves to block out and numb the pain?

In some cultures, grief is experienced through wailing: letting out the energy and releasing it to the universe. We, on the other hand, tend to sit quietly in our grief. Are we too afraid to share our most vulnerable and human side? In so doing, we risk denying ourselves what we want most: human connection in the midst of deep sorrow.

Sugar, sugar—everywhere sugar

My father's eightieth birthday celebration fell during Passover. Immediate family members flew in from all parts of the country. My mom hosted the second Seder at their house, though we all wanted to spare my mom the burden of preparing for this awesome feast and complicated menu. To help her get ready, I began a hunt for catering options from local health-food stores.

I found one proprietor happy to work with me. I asked for side dishes without sugar for my diabetic father and one that fit a vegan diet for my sister (no animal products, including dairy or eggs). *Seven hundred* recipes later, the deli manager finally came up with two that fit the bill.

She easily met the vegan request for my sister. But finding savory food without added sweetness for my father wasn't as easy. And this was a *health*-food store.

I'm both amazed and appalled. You can find sugar (if you look) in "healthy" mayonnaise under the guise of brown rice syrup or in tomato sauce or in "healthy" cheese slices or in soy milk under a variety of aliases.

Are even the health-food stores buying into mainstream American issues of adding sugar to everything as a filler or taste-enhancer? Or a substitute for healthful spices and condiments? Or is it as one food manufacturing executive said, "We're only giving you what the public wants"? Are we afraid to actually taste the real taste of food? Is there such a lack of taste in foods that we need to spruce up every brussel sprout and green bean? I don't think so. Do an experiment, next time you go to a restaurant, ask to see their ingredient list. Check to see if there is any item savory or sweet that does not have sugar in it. Sugar ingested stimulates a desire for more sugar. Here's another tip—all the nutrients your body gets from fruit is available in vegetables minus the sugar.

Children's eating habits and parental responsibility

Where does parental responsibility end and a child's right to choose begin?

We don't let children drive cars until they are sixteen. The government has decided that before that age, children would be more of a hazard to themselves and others. In Compassionate or Nonviolent Communication, we may consider this a way to protect our children from harm.

Children also are limited in their ability to drink legally in a bar until they turn eighteen or twenty-one, depending on the state in which you live. This, too, is done to protect them and others from harm.

What kind of responsibility do parents have for protecting their children through the foods they serve and provide for their children? Do you spend more time researching the type of computer or toy to buy than what nutrients are found in the food you are feeding your children?

Think about it ...

- Do you allow your children to drink unlimited amounts of fruit juice or soda?

- Do you limit their ice cream, candy bar, and cookie intake?

- Do you provide a variety of fruits and vegetables for your children, giving them the nutrients their bodies need to grow strong and healthy?

- Do you provide protein foods and foods high in magnesium for energy and strength?

- Do you read the labels of food items you buy in the store to ensure the highest-quality products for their health?

- Does the issue of providing tasty foods that contribute to health constitute protection and not punishment?

I worry that allowing your child to drink and eat foods with artificial colorings, hydrogenation, and high sugar content is poisoning them. I know of children who, by seven years of age, already have three crowns in their mouth. Is anyone saying *no* to their requests for sugary snacks and protecting them from harming themselves? Recently, doctors found Type 2 diabetes in children as young as five, and heart disease in twelve-year-olds.

Do you want your children to outlive you? This won't happen unless parents and guardians in our culture drastically change the way they feed their children—and support them in exercising their bodies.

If you had a magic wand and granted me three wishes for you and your family's nutritional well-being, these would be my wishes:

1. If your children are soda drinkers, allow soda only on occasion—once per month maximum. (Make it sugared rather than diet soda and preferably one with cane sugar, or better yet, stevia, or xylitol.) Our bodies need water.
2. Substitute foods with hydrogenated oils with trans-fat-free varieties like olive oil, butter, ghee, coconut oil, sesame oil, and lard.
3. Provide your children with sweets made from stevia, xylitol, lucuma, or palm sugar. It's easier on the blood sugar and bakes similar to regular sugar, or make a raw dessert with cashews, cacao nibs, and stevia.

Are you willing to do something about this crisis, starting with your own family?

You as a parent are on the front lines of this issue. You have the power to help your children with choices that will support their health and well-being—moment by moment *and* for a lifetime.

School lunch programs and a school's responsibility
What is the responsibility of the school?

How many schools in the United States provide candy, soda, and chip-filled vending machines and serve brand-name fast foods? What kind of impact does easy access to these less-than-nutritious foods have on students' abilities to learn and be present?

When Dr. Ehrenfried Pfeiffer asked Rudolf Steiner, philosopher and founder of the Waldorf school movement, why people today appear unable to develop and act according to all they've learned and seem to know, Steiner replied, "This is a problem of nutrition."

Worldwide, Waldorf schools make a conscious effort to keep school snacks and meals as natural as possible. Most schools have a garden. They encourage students to learn how to grow vegetables and grind grain. Salads, fruits, nuts, and simple soups are Waldorf's staples.

What a difference from schools whose after-school activities are sponsored by the Coca-Cola Company! Is it possible these schools are more worried about school funding than the harm caused by drinking thirteen teaspoons of sugar in every can?

Let's focus on needs for a moment. My guess is that everyone's needs can be met. Surely there are ways to fund school programs without hurting the health of children.

What about Coca-Cola's needs? Is it about their need for visibility? Contribution? Must they satisfy those needs at the expense of children? Aren't there other ways to gain visibility? To contribute to causes they deem worthy? With their vast creativity and marketing know-how, what if they invented a product that enhances health instead of destroying it?

If you want inspiration—and share my desire to transform school lunch programs for the health and learning of our students—check out the fifteen-minute DVD offered by Natural Ovens Bakery (ordering information in the subsequent resources section). Highlighted in the film *Super Size Me*, this DVD shows the impact of fresh, healthful foods on learning and behavior, based on a five-year study at an alternative high school in Wisconsin.

Make copies of it, show it to your friends and neighbors, and bring healthful food to schools in your area. Check out Jamie Oliver's Food Revolution at jamieoliver.com. He is helping to change school lunch programs one school, one community at a time. You can help restore our children's health and well-being—indeed, their very future.

The Beginning

"If you have the courage to begin,
you have the courage to succeed."
DAVID VISCOTT

Information is alive. It expands to fit our evolving curiosities. It extends beyond the pages we capture it on. Nutritional information, especially, has a tendency to change with every new research study, as I explored in my "soapbox" section. I've done my best to bring you what I know now. Tomorrow I may know better. I resonate with what Maya Angelou told Oprah Winfrey, "You did then what you knew then; when you knew better, you did better."

This applies to you, too. Although we're close to the end of this book, it's the beginning of your journey. Eating by choice is not only a process, it's a celebration, it's a movement: You're off to witness your eating habits with fresh eyes, renewed sensuality, and a deep and growing love for your body.

In Compassionate Communication, you recognize the moment of choice before reacting, responding, and communicating when someone else's words or actions may trigger you. So, too, with eating. You recognize the choice at any moment by stopping, tuning in, and choosing what step or action to take next, based on your needs in the moment. You listen to and engage with what is alive and present in you, rather than burying it under rote behavior.

Now you know that habits are simply behaviors we do over and over again with little or no consciousness. With your awakened consciousness, may you make choices that meet your needs. May you choose to find friendship with food, allowing the nutrients to nourish your body. And may you choose to have the kind of relationship with food that you would most enjoy. Above all, may you learn to explore food and eating with acceptance, playfulness, and compassion.

Here's to choice in all we do,

Sylvia

A Buffet of Resources
Maintaining Consciousness

"Everyone who has ever taken a shower has had an idea. It's the person who gets out of the shower, dries off, and does something about it that makes a difference."

NOLAN BUSHNELL

When you are conscious, you're aware of your emotional needs. From this consciousness, you may ask yourself how many calories and what food groups will contribute to your body's needs for nourishment and optimal functioning. How much do you actually need to maintain, lose, or gain weight—or whatever it is you want to do?

An abundance of books, websites, and associations exist to guide you in your health and wellness journey. To find the right match for you, check out your chosen resource with your body, too. Your body knows. Does your chest tighten? Do you feel a glitch in your gut? Or does your heart open? Do you feel relaxed? How is your breathing? Remember, you are your own best authority.

Recipe favorites

When I decide to make changes in my eating choices, I find it helpful to have recipes handy that will launch me on my way. For some fun, tasty foods that will nourish your body and honor your desire for something new in your life, you're invited to visit: *www.EatByChoice.com* where you'll find these recipes and more:

- Steel Cut Oats and More
- Vegetable Burro/Burrito
- Peanut butter cookies
- Quick/Easy Hummus
- Mediterranean Medley Salad
- Israeli/Arab Vegetable Salad
- Yam/Yukon Gold Potato Bake
- Carob goddess cake
- Lemon/Poppy Seed Cookies
- Carob/Walnut Clusters

Books and other resources I've found especially helpful

Live in the Balance, The Ground-Breaking East-West Nutrition Program by Linda Prout, Marlowe & Company, 2000.

Own Your Health: Choosing the Best from Alternative & Conventional Medicine by Roanne Weisman, with Brian Berman, M.D., Health Communications, 2003.

The pH Miracle: Balance Your Diet, Reclaim Your Health by Robert O. Young, Ph.D., and Shelley Redford Young, Warner Books, 2002.

Guide to Healthy Restaurant Eating by Hope Warshaw, M.M.Sc., R.D., C.D.E., American Diabetes Association, 2002, second edition.

Nourishing Traditions: The Cookbook That Challenges Politically Correct Nutrition and the Diet Dictocrats by Sally Fallon, with Mary G. Enig, Ph.D., New Trends Publishing, 1999, second edition.

How to Get Your Kid to Eat—But Not Too Much by Ellyn Satter, Bull Publishing Co., 1987.

The Path of Least Resistance: Learning to Become the Creative Force in Your Own Life by Robert Fritz, Ballantine Books, 1989.

French Women Don't Get Fat: The Secret of Eating for Pleasure by Mireille Guiliano, Chatto & Windus, 2005.

Healing Our Planet, Healing Ourselves: The Power to Change Within to Change the World, edited by Dawson Church and Geralyn Gendreau, Elite Books, 2004, 2005.

Omnivore's Dilemma, A Natural History of Four Meals by Michael Pollan, Penguin Press, 2007.

Animal, Vegetable, Miracle, A Year of Food Life by Barbara Kingsolver, HarperCollins, 2007.

Mindless Eating, Why We Eat More Than We Think by Brian Wansink, Ph.D., Bantam Books, 2006.

Full Moon Feast, Food and the Hunger for Connection by Jessica Prentice, Chelsea Green Publishing, 2006.

Vegetarian Cooking for Everyone by Deborah Madison, Broadway Books, 1997.

Additional resources

Dr. Joseph Mercola, *www.mercola.com*

"For cutting edge information about REAL health products and information on living well, Dr. Mercola's site is an essential to all who are yearing to be balanced. His studies and products have been a staple in my life."

—Mariel Hemingway

Weston A. Price Foundation

"Nutrition for Living Shopping Guide: Finding the Healthiest Foods in Supermarkets and Health Food Stores"
Telephone: 202-333-HEAL (4325) or *www.westonaprice.org*
The foundation has other free booklets on cancer prevention, soy alert, cholesterol, milk, hydrogenated fats, and more. You also can join the organization and receive regular newsletters.

Nutrition for Optimal Health Association (NOHA)

P.O. Box 380
Winnetka, IL 60093
www.nutrition4health.org
Telephone: 847-60HEALTH (847-604-3258)

Natural Ovens Bakery

Manitowoc, Wisconsin
"Appleton Alternative High School: Impact of Fresh, Healthy Foods on Learning and Behavior—A 5-Year Study" (15 minutes), 2004.

To purchase this DVD contact:
Website: *www.naturalovens.com*
Toll-free telephone: 800-558-3535
Make copies of the DVD, show it to your friends and neighbors, and bring healthful food to schools in your

area. You can help restore our children's health, well-being, and their very future.

HeartMath and Compassionate Communication (NVC)

Some people have found Compassionate Communication and HeartMath a powerful combination. To learn more about HeartMath, check out *www.heartmath.org.*

Food and body counseling/nutritional support

Becky Coleman, Ph.D., founder of Taking Your Own Shape™, offers groundbreaking classes, workshops, retreats, and individual mentoring sessions for women and men of all sizes seeking healthy relationship with body, soul, food, and weight.

Website: *www.o-c-e-a-n.com*
Email: becky@o-c-e-a-n.com
Telephone: 562-595-2885

Linda Prout, M.S., nutritionist extraordinaire, is a consultant, speaker, author, and counselor to individuals seeking more energy and greater health. Together, we offer teleseminars—meeting our emotional needs and the needs of our bodies at the same time. Linda offers phone appointments and email consultations, chock full of helpful information. You can receive her Top Nutrition Tips by email. Register on her website:

www.lindaprout.com
Email: linda@lindaprout.com

Laurel Inman, is a professional life coach that specializes in helping people break free from the cycles of emotional eating and food addiction. Laurel's programs help people acquire peace and freedom with food and weight issues. Her approach, called Fire Your Diet, connects people with the natural hunger cycles of their body. This type of education eliminates the dependence on dieting and portion control, which naturally leads to long term success.

Website: *www.lifecatalyst.net*
(Intentional Eating Forum)
Email: laurel@laurelinman.com
Telephone: 520-292-1209

Tasty tips

[Adapted from "A Rainbow of Vitamin-Packed Choices" by Mary Beth Faller, *The Arizona Republic*, February 22, 2005, and the Produce for Better Health Foundation]

One way to know you're getting the balance of nutrients from your fruits and vegetables is to add color to your diet. For greater health, choose one from each color every day.

Blue/Purple: blueberries, plums, prunes, raisins, eggplant, red cabbage
Improves urinary tract health and contains antiaging antioxidants.

Green: avocados, green grapes, honeydew, pears, limes, asparagus, broccoli, green onions, spinach, zucchini, snow peas, kiwi

Helps prevent some birth defects, maintains strong bones and teeth, and gives you energy.

White: bananas, cauliflower, garlic, ginger, mushrooms, onions, potatoes, white corn

Maintains cholesterol levels for optimal health, lowers risk of some cancers.

Yellow/orange: peaches, pineapples, butternut squash, carrots, yellow peppers, yellow potatoes, pumpkins, rutabagas, sweet potatoes, apricots, cantaloupe, grapefruit, lemons, mangoes, oranges, papayas *Improves vision health, boosts immune system.*

Red: red apples, cherries, cranberries, red grapes, pink or red grapefruit, red pears, raspberries, strawberries, red watermelon, beets, red peppers, radishes, red onions, red potatoes, tomatoes, pomegranates, rhubarb. *Maintains heart health, boosts memory function.*

Fun tidbits

If you are constipated, in addition to drinking water, eating fiber and exercising, try adding one to two tablespoons per day of flax seed oil or cod liver oil to your diet.

Purchase organic extra virgin cold pressed olive oil in a dark container and store it away from the stove to maintain optimum nutritional value.

Hydrogenated fats tend to be stored in the belly, close to your heart. Choose healthful fats like olive oil, grass fed butter, ghee, sesame oil, or coconut oil.

When using fresh ginger, grate whole unpeeled ginger onto a cutting board. Take the ginger shavings and squeeze it into your recipe before serving. You will have no ginger pieces just the flavor of ginger.

Ten ways to cut sugar cravings

[Reprinted with permission from Linda Prout's *Live in the Balance: The Ground-Breaking East-West Nutrition Program*]

Most people consider sugar a healthful food. The problem is just how to stop yearning for those chocolates, jelly beans, and brownies. The following steps will actually reduce your desire for sweets by altering the chemistry of your blood and brain, including stabilizing blood sugar and stimulating serotonin and other brain chemicals that keep you content without a cookie. Many of these dietary principles are part of the Chinese way of life.

1. Have a nonsweet breakfast containing a protein-rich food. Choose a whole grain plus the appropriate protein source for your body: eggs, lox, smoked fish, lean poultry sausage, soy products, beans, nuts, or seeds.

2. Include adequate, high-quality protein at lunch. Again, choose the protein-rich foods best for your body: eggs, fish, poultry, lean beef or pork, nuts, seeds, or legumes.

3. Avoid excess raw fruits, raw vegetables, and juice. (Fruits and especially juices are high in sugars, which can leave your blood sugar low and create a desire for more sweets.) Raw fruits and vegetables also are energetically very "cooling" in Eastern nutrition, a quality that can drive up your desire for food that is "warming," such as sugar.

4. Include cooked leafy greens daily, especially if chocolate cravings are a problem.

5. Drink green tea daily. It helps to maintain stable blood-sugar levels, thereby minimizing cravings for sugar.

6. Avoid artificial sweeteners. Your body may respond as if they are real sugars.

7. Bite the bullet and reduce or eliminate refined sugars (sucrose, fructose, fruit juice, honey, and syrups).

8. Get adequate, full-spectrum lighting. Natural light is essential for the brain to produce serotonin, the calming brain chemical that prevents sugar cravings. Take a twenty-minute walk outdoors in the early morning, sit near a bright window, or use full-spectrum lighting in your workspace.

9. Include an essential-fat source, such as flax, pumpkin, or hemp seed oils, or the omega-3 fatty acids DHA and EPA present in fish oils.

10. Try supplements of magnesium (350 to 500 mg) and chromium (200 to 500 mcg), minerals that stabilize

blood sugar, or the herbs *gymnema sylvestre* or fennel leaf, or licorice root. (Licorice root tastes sweet, plus it stimulates the adrenals, which can boost energy in someone with weak adrenals. In large amounts, licorice may raise blood pressure, however, and should be used with caution.)

Conscious-eating exercise: Practice presence with your dining experience

After you have prepared a plate of food, sit down and commit the first five minutes to practicing conscious consumption. The purpose of this exercise is to notice

> *"One of the very nicest things about life is the way we must regularly stop whatever it is we are doing and devote our attention to eating."*
> LUCIANO PAVAROTTI,
> from his book *Pavarotti, My Own Story*

what foods you enjoy and why you enjoy them. It's also about taking the time to chew your food and savor the sensuousness of the experience. Trust your body's inner knowing.

Put a forkful or spoonful of food into your mouth. Close your eyes. Notice the taste, texture, temperature, and mouth feel. Are you enjoying what you taste? Are the textures pleasing to you?

Chew slowly. Relish what's in your mouth. When you have completely chewed that bite, open your eyes and try another with a different food sensation on your fork. Put the bite in your mouth and close your eyes. Again notice. Repeat this exercise for five minutes or until you are satisfied with the experiment. You may find that food you had enjoyed will have less appeal, and other foods will increase their appeal. This is part of the food-awakening experience.

Take your time ... Notice ... Enjoy ... Savor!

Compassionate Communication recap

First, figure out what a particular person said or did that stimulated feelings in you, then tune in to how you feel. Feelings happen somewhere in your body. When they happen in your head, you're likely still in judgment mode and not connected to your underlying feelings.

Then uncover what your need or needs are related to this incident. All human beings share the same needs, which is what connects us.

After you've uncovered your needs, make a positive, doable request.

Requests are about asking for something back from the other person in this moment, or of yourself.

A request may start with "Are you willing to tell me ..."

Or "How do you feel about ..."

You don't ask people not to do something. It would be difficult for someone to "do a don't," so ask for what you do want in a doable way. You also will not want your request to be vague because you won't know if your request is satisfied.

An example of this is, "I want you to understand me."

How will you know unless you ask for a specific doable request?

You may want to say, "Can you tell me what you heard so I can see if I was clear and understood?"

The second part of this process is listening with empathy.

The four steps are the same, only now we are hearing the other person's message.

It may sound like this: "When you said you didn't want to go out to eat tonight, was it because you're feeling exhausted and sad? Are you wanting/needing down time? Would you like me to make dinner for us instead?"

When you listen with empathy, it does not mean that it works for you to make dinner. You are tuning in to the other person's world without putting your own agenda into the equation.

If it doesn't work for you to make dinner, and this is what your partner would like, then you speak your truth with honesty, which may sound like this: "When I hear that you want me to cook dinner, I feel overwhelmed and exhausted as well. I would like to find an option that works for both of us. Would it work for you if I ordered takeout?"

Normal eating

[From the handout Ellyn Satter gives to people whose eating issues she treats. Reprinted with permission from Ellyn Satter.]

Normal eating is essentially positive and flexible eating that depends on internal cues to regulate it.

Normal eating is being able to eat when you are hungry and continue eating until you are satisfied. It is being able to choose food you like and eat it and truly get enough of it— not just stop eating because you think you should. Normal eating is being able to use some moderate constraint in your food selection to get the right food, but not being so restrictive that you miss out on pleasurable foods.

Normal eating is giving yourself permission to eat sometimes because you are happy, sad, or bored—or just because it feels good. Normal eating is three meals a day most of the time, but it can also be choosing to munch along. It is leaving some cookies on the plate because you know you can have some again tomorrow, or it is eating more now because they taste so wonderful when they are fresh. Normal eating is overeating at times: feeling satisfied and uncomfortable. It is also undereating at times and wishing you had more.

Normal eating is trusting your body to make up for your mistakes in eating. Normal eating takes up some of your time and attention but keeps its place as only one important area of your life. In short, normal eating is flexible. It varies in response to your emotions, your schedule, your hunger, and your proximity to food.

Without outside influences, babies eat normally. They take in food and regulate it without a lot of outside influences disrupting that ability.

Gentle reminders

- Without compassion, change is impossible.
- Tune in: How do you feel? What do you need?
- Eating is often a strategy to meet needs other than physical hunger; consider other strategies as well.
- Notice how you feel after you take your first bite and after you eat a meal. Are you satisfied?
- Did you enjoy it? Did it meet your physical and aesthetic needs?
- Practice choice in all you do.

Request for Stories

If you have changed your relationship with food and your body and want to share your story, I would like to hear it. Feel free to also request future books on specific topics connected to health, nutrition, and NVC. For the most updated information, go to our website at eatbychoice.net. Please send to *silgiraffe@gmail.com*. I look forward to hearing from you.

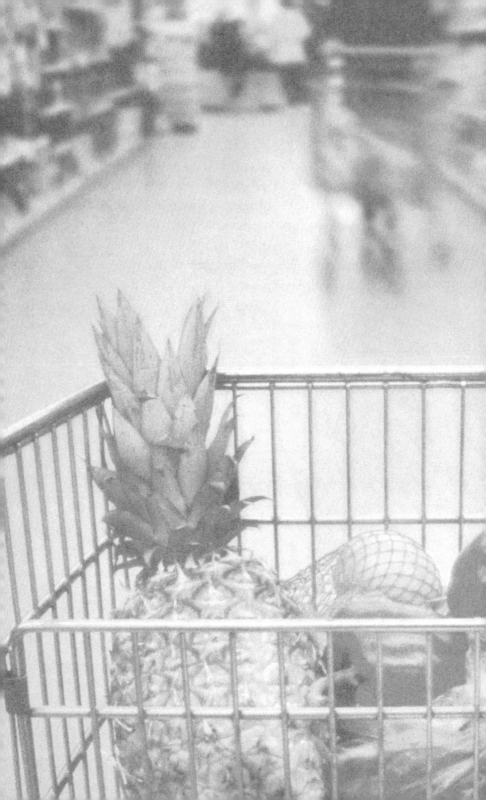

Index

coronary heart disease
(CHD), 72–73
Cousens, Gabriel, 75
cravings, 17–22, 64, 90–91
crunchy foods, anxiety and,
12
cultural influences on eating
habits, 24–30, 44

D

death of sibling, eating
disorders and, 74
dehydration, mistaken for
hunger, 45, 48
Delany, Richard, 69, 72
demand/resistance cycle, 8–9,
16, 28, 33, 35, 61
demand vs. request, 61
see also requests
deprivation, 8
diabetes, 10, 69, 84
diet change, effect on
students, 27
dieting, 8–11
digestive problems, 41
Downey, Robert, Jr., 36

E

eating disorders
autonomy needs and, 27
grieving and, 74–75
see also emotional eating;
overeating
edible substitutes for needs,
6, 11–13, 45

email address, author's, 97
emotional eating, 6, 11–14,
21–22, 25, 45–47
see also addiction to food;
food cravings
empathy, for others, 31, 93–94
see also self-empathy
enjoying food fully, 7, 18,
37–38, 92–93
exercise
for conscious-eating,
92–93
physical, 52–53
expressing feelings and
needs, 60–62, 65

F

fad diets, 9–11
Faller, Mary Beth, 88
Fallon, Sally, 85
fast food, 25–26, 27, 55,
79–80
fats, dietary, 67–73
FDA (US Food and Drug
Administration), 68–71
feelings
avoidance of, 74–75
connection to, 7, 11, 17,
21–22, 60–61, 93
elicited by food, 40
expressing, 60–62, 65
list of, 109
managing with food,
11–14, 19, 21–22, 25,
45–47

T

taste appeal of food, 41–44
Tasty tips, 88–89
Ten Ways to cut sugar cravings, 90–92
"Think Thin, Be Thin" (Helmering and Hales), 47
thirst, mistaken for hunger, 45, 48
trans fats, 67–73
translating messages of others with NVC, 30–34
travel, healthy eating strategies for, 55–58
Traveling Mercies: Some Thoughts on Faith, Lamott, 13, 36
Tucker, Susan, 52
tuning in to feelings and needs, 13–18, 21–22, 81–82, 95
see also awareness; feelings; needs
Type 2 diabetes, 10, 68–69, 78

U

urinary-tract infections, 19
US Department of Agriculture (USDA), 68

V

vegetables, 11, 20, 32, 33, 42, 43, 45, 49, 56, 57, 76, 77, 79, 88, 91

Vegetarian Cooking for Everyone, Madison, 85
vending machines, 55, 79–80

W

Waldorf schools, 79
Warshaw, Hope, 84
water, need for, 45, 48
weight loss difficulties
effect of cultural influences on, 24–25
receiving support from others, 63–64
supporting others, 59–65
see also obesity
Weisman, Roanne, 20
Weston A. Price Foundation, 86
white foods, nutritional value, 89–91
Williamson, Marianne, 60
Winfrey, Oprah, 10, 36, 50

X

xylitol, 78

Y

yeast overgrowth, 20
yellow foods, nutritional value, 88–89
yogurt, 19, 20, 34, 43
Young, Robert O., 19, 84
Young, Shelley Redford, 19, 84
yo-yo dieting, 10

The Four-Part Nonviolent Communication Process

Clearly expressing
how **I am**
without blaming
or criticizing

Empathically receiving
how **you are**
without hearing
blame or criticism

OBSERVATIONS

1. What I observe *(see, hear, remember, imagine, free from my evaluations)* that does or does not contribute to my well-being:

   "When I (see, hear) . . . "

1. What you observe *(see, hear, remember, imagine, free from your evaluations)* that does or does not contribute to your well-being:

   "When you see/hear . . . "

   (Sometimes unspoken when offering empathy)

FEELINGS

2. How I feel *(emotion or sensation rather than thought)* in relation to what I observe:

   "I feel . . . "

2. How you feel *(emotion or sensation rather than thought)* in relation to what you observe:

   "You feel . . ."

NEEDS

3. What I need or value *(rather than a preference, or a specific action)* that causes my feelings:

   " . . . because I need/value . . . "

3. What you need or value *(rather than a preference, or a specific action)* that causes your feelings:

   " . . . because you need/value . . ."

Clearly requesting that
which would enrich **my**
life without demanding

Empathically receiving that
which would enrich **your** life
without hearing any demand

REQUESTS

4. The concrete actions I would like taken:

   "Would you be willing to . . . ?"

4. The concrete actions you would like taken:

   "Would you like . . . ?"

   (Sometimes unspoken when offering empathy)

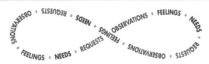

Some Basic Feelings We All Have

Feelings when needs are fulfilled

- Amazed
- Comfortable
- Confident
- Eager
- Energetic
- Fulfilled
- Glad
- Hopeful
- Inspired
- Intrigued
- Joyous
- Moved
- Optimistic
- Proud
- Relieved
- Stimulated
- Surprised
- Thankful
- Touched
- Trustful

Feelings when needs are not fulfilled

- Angry
- Annoyed
- Concerned
- Confused
- Disappointed
- Discouraged
- Distressed
- Embarrassed
- Frustrated
- Helpless
- Hopeless
- Impatient
- Irritated
- Lonely
- Nervous
- Overwhelmed
- Puzzled
- Reluctant
- Sad
- Uncomfortable

Some Basic Needs We All Have

Autonomy
- Choosing dreams/goals/values
- Choosing plans for fulfilling one's dreams, goals, values

Celebration
- Celebrating the creation of life and dreams fulfilled
- Celebrating losses: loved ones, dreams, etc. (mourning)

Integrity
- Authenticity • Creativity
- Meaning • Self-worth

Interdependence
- Acceptance • Appreciation
- Closeness • Community
- Consideration
- Contribution to the enrichment of life
- Emotional Safety • Empathy

Physical Nurturance
- Air • Food
- Movement, exercise
- Protection from life-threatening forms of life: viruses, bacteria, insects, predatory animals
- Rest • Sexual Expression
- Shelter • Touch • Water

Play
- Fun • Laughter

Spiritual Communion
- Beauty • Harmony
- Inspiration • Order • Peace
- Honesty (the empowering honesty that enables us to learn from our limitations)
- Love • Reassurance
- Respect • Support
- Trust • Understanding

About PuddleDancer Press

PuddleDancer Press (PDP) is the premier publisher of Nonviolent Communication™ related works. Its mission is to provide high-quality materials to help people create a world in which all needs are met compassionately. Publishing revenues are used to develop new books, and implement promotion campaigns for NVC and Marshall Rosenberg. By working in partnership with the Center for Nonviolent Communication and NVC trainers, teams, and local supporters, PDP has created a comprehensive promotion effort that has helped bring NVC to thousands of new people each year.

Since 2003 PDP has donated more than 60,000 NVC books to organizations, decision-makers, and individuals in need around the world. This program is supported in part by donations made to CNVC and by partnerships with like-minded organizations around the world.

Visit the PDP website at www.NonviolentCommunication.com to find the following resources:

- **Shop NVC**—Continue your learning. Purchase our NVC titles online safely, affordably, and conveniently. Find everyday discounts on individual titles, multiple-copies, and book packages. Learn more about our authors and read endorsements of NVC from world-renowned communication experts and peacemakers. www.NonviolentCommunication.com/store/

- **NVC Quick Connect e-Newsletter**—Sign up today to receive our monthly e-Newsletter, filled with expert articles, upcoming training opportunities with our authors, and exclusive specials on NVC learning materials. Archived e-Newsletters are also available

- **About NVC**—Learn more about these life-changing communication and conflict resolution skills including an overview of the NVC process, key facts about NVC, and more.

- **About Marshall Rosenberg**—Access press materials, biography, and more about this world-renowned peacemaker, educator, bestselling author, and founder of the Center for Nonviolent Communication.

- **Free Resources for Learning NVC**—Find free weekly tips series, NVC article archive, and other great resources to make learning these vital communication skills just a little easier.

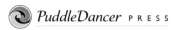

For more information, please contact PuddleDancer Press at:

2240 Encinitas Blvd., Ste. D-911 • Encinitas, CA 92024
Phone: 760-652-5754 • Fax: 760-274-6400
Email: email@puddledancer.com • www.NonviolentCommunication.com

About the Center for Nonviolent Communication

The Center for Nonviolent Communication (CNVC) is an international nonprofit peacemaking organization whose vision is a world where everyone's needs are met peacefully. CNVC is devoted to supporting the spread of Nonviolent Communication (NVC) around the world.

Founded in 1984 by Dr. Marshall B. Rosenberg, CNVC has been contributing to a vast social transformation in thinking, speaking and acting— showing people how to connect in ways that inspire compassionate results. NVC is now being taught around the globe in communities, schools, prisons, mediation centers, churches, businesses, professional conferences, and more. More than 200 certified trainers and hundreds more teach NVC to approximately 250,000 people each year in 35 countries.

CNVC believes that NVC training is a crucial step to continue building a compassionate, peaceful society. Your tax-deductible donation will help CNVC continue to provide training in some of the most impoverished, violent corners of the world. It will also support the development and continuation of organized projects aimed at bringing NVC training to high-need geographic regions and populations.

To make a tax-deductible donation or to learn more about the valuable resources described below, visit the CNVC website at www.CNVC.org:

- **Training and Certification**—Find local, national, and international training opportunities, access trainer certification information, connect to local NVC communities, trainers, and more.

- **CNVC Bookstore**—Find mail or phone order information for a complete selection of NVC books, booklets, audio, and video materials at the CNVC website.

- **CNVC Projects**—Seven regional and theme-based projects provide focus and leadership for teaching NVC in a particular application or geographic region.

- **E-Groups and List Servs**—Join one of several moderated, topic-based NVC e-groups and list servs developed to support individual learning and the continued growth of NVC worldwide.

For more information, please contact CNVC at:

5600-A San Francisco Rd., NE, Albuquerque, NM 87109
Ph: 505-244-4041 • Fax: 505-247-0414
Email: cnvc@CNVC.org • Website: www.CNVC.org

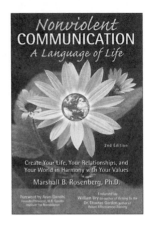

Nonviolent Communication:
A Language of Life, Second Edition

*Create Your Life, Your Relationships, and
Your World in Harmony With Your Values*

Marshall B. Rosenberg, Ph.D.

$19.95 — Trade Paper 6x9, 240pp
ISBN: 978-1-892005-03-8

Most of us are hungry for skills to improve the quality of our relationships, to deepen our sense of personal empowerment or to simply communicate more effectively. In this internationally acclaimed text, Marshall Rosenberg offers insightful stories, anecdotes, practical exercises, and role-plays that will literally change your approach to communication for the better. Discover how the language you use can strengthen your relationships, build trust, prevent conflicts, and heal pain. Revolutionary, yet simple, NVC offers the most effective tools to reduce violence and create peace—one interaction at a time.

More than 800,000 copies of this landmark book have been sold. Printed in twenty-five languages around the globe.

"Unless, as grandfather would say, 'we become the change we wish to see in the world,' no change will ever take place . . . If we change ourselves we can change the world, and changing ourselves begins with changing our language and methods of communication. I highly recommend reading this book and applying the Nonviolent Communication process it teaches."

> **—Foreword by Arun Gandhi**, grandson of Mahatma Gandhi and
> co-founder of the M.K. Gandhi Institute for Nonviolence

"Nonviolent communication is a simple yet powerful methodology for communicating in a way that meets both parties' needs. This is one of the most useful books you will ever read."

> **—William Ury**, coauthor of *Getting to Yes* and author of *The Third Side*

"I believe the principles and techniques in this book can literally change the world, but more importantly, they can change the quality of your life with your spouse, your children, your neighbors, your co-workers, and everyone else you interact with."

> **—Jack Canfield**, author, *Chicken Soup for the Soul*

Available from PuddleDancer Press, the Center for Nonviolent Communication, all major bookstores, and Amazon.com. Distributed by Independent Publisher's Group: 800-888-4741.

SAVE 10% at NonviolentCommunication.com with coupon code: **bookads**

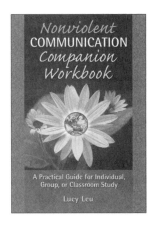

Nonviolent Communication Companion Workbook

A Practical Guide for Individual, Group, or Classroom Study

by Lucy Leu

$21.95 — Trade Paper 7x10, 224pp
ISBN: 978-1-892005-04-5

Learning Nonviolent Communication has often been equated with learning a whole new language. The *NVC Companion Workbook* helps you put these powerful, effective skills into practice with chapter-by-chapter study of Marshall Rosenberg's cornerstone text, *NVC: A Language of Life.*

An exceptional resource for:

- **Individuals**—Integrate the liberating practice of the NVC process in your daily life as the workbook guides you through self-directed study.

- **Group Practice**—Find structured guidance for practice facilitation including group-process suggestions, customizable activities, and ideas for handling common group challenges.

- **Educators**—Find everything you need to develop your own NVC course or augment any existing curriculum, including an extensive reference and resource section.

"I've used this workbook now in two prison facilities. It has been a wonderful tool for men and women who are committed to gaining useful life skills in some of the toughest of environments."

> **—Karen Campbell**, workforce and lifeskills coordinator,
> Coffee Creek Corrections Facility

"We went over real-life situations and followed various exercises that promoted understanding the content more fully. This practice was the key for my success in understanding and using NVC!"

> **—Kirsten Ingram**, finance and administration officer,
> Children's Commission Province of British Columbia

Available from PuddleDancer Press, the Center for Nonviolent Communication, all major bookstores, and Amazon.com. Distributed by Independent Publisher's Group: 800-888-4741.

SAVE 10% at NonviolentCommunication.com with coupon code: **bookads**

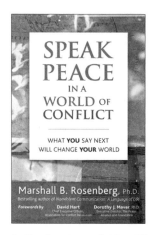

Speak Peace in a World of Conflict

What You Say Next Will Change Your World

by Marshall B. Rosenberg, Ph.D.

$15.95 — Trade Paper 5-3/8x8-3/8, 208pp
ISBN: 978-1-892005-17-5

In every interaction, every conversation, and in every thought, you have a choice—to promote peace or perpetuate violence. International peacemaker, mediator, and healer, Dr. Marshall Rosenberg shows you how the language you use is the key to enriching life. Take the first step to reduce violence, heal pain, resolve conflicts, and spread peace on our planet—by developing an internal consciousness of peace rooted in the language you use each day.

Speak Peace is filled with inspiring stories, lessons, and ideas drawn from more than forty years of mediating conflicts and healing relationships in some of the most war-torn, impoverished, and violent corners of the world. *Speak Peace* offers insight, practical skills, and powerful tools that will profoundly change your relationships and the course of your life for the better.

Bestselling author of the internationally acclaimed,
Nonviolent Communication: A Language of Life

Discover how you can create an internal consciousness of peace as the first step toward effective personal, professional, and social change. Find complete chapters on the mechanics of Speaking Peace, conflict resolution, transforming business culture, transforming enemy images, addressing terrorism, transforming authoritarian structures, expressing and receiving gratitude, and social change.

"*Speak Peace* is a book that comes at an appropriate time when anger and violence dominates human attitudes. Marshall Rosenberg gives us the means to create peace through our speech and communication. A brilliant book."
   —Arun Gandhi, president, M. K. Gandhi Institute for Nonviolence, USA

"*Speak Peace* sums up decades of healing and peacework. It would be hard to list all the kinds of people who can benefit from reading this book, because it's really any and all of us."
   —Dr. Michael Nagler, author, *America Without Violence* and
   Is There No Other Way: A Search for a Nonviolent Future

Available from PuddleDancer Press, the Center for Nonviolent Communication, all major bookstores, and Amazon.com. Distributed by Independent Publisher's Group: 800-888-4741.

Being Genuine

Stop Being Nice, Start Being Real

by Thomas d'Ansembourg

$17.95 — Trade Paper 5-3/8x8-3/8, 280pp
ISBN: 978-1-892005-21-2

Being Genuine brings Thomas d'Ansembourg's blockbuster French title to the English market. His work offers you a fresh new perspective on the proven skills offered in the bestselling book, *Nonviolent Communication: A Language of Life.* Drawing on his own real-life examples and stories, d'Ansembourg provides practical skills and concrete steps that allow us to safely remove the masks we wear, which prevent the intimacy and satisfaction we desire with our intimate partners, children, parents, friends, family, and colleagues.

With this Fresh, New Perspective on Communication, Learn to:
- Safely remove the masks we hide behind
- Overcome past prejudices and conditioned beliefs
- Purge your thinking and language of anything that generates conflict
- Accept responsibility for your feelings and actions
- Transform the fears that block us from connecting with others
- Create the space you need to connect with loved ones or colleagues
- Practice unconditional love each day

"Here is further proof, if any were needed, of the effectiveness of Nonviolent Communication in improving human relationships at nearly any level."
—Dr. Michael Nagler, author, *America Without Violence* and *Is There No Other Way?*

"Through this book, we can feel Nonviolent Communication not as a formula but as a rich, meaningful way of life, both intellectually and emotionally."
—Vicki Robin, co-founder, Conversation Cafes, coauthor, *Your Money or Your Life*

Based on Marshall Rosenberg's Nonviolent Communication process

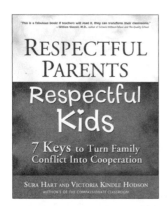

Respectful Parents, Respectful Kids

7 Keys to Turn Family Conflict Into Co-operation

Sura Hart and Victoria Kindle Hodson

$17.95 – Trade Paper 7.5x9.25, 256pp
ISBN: 978-1-892005-22-9

Stop the Struggle

Find the Co-operation and Mutual Respect You Want!

Do more than simply correct bad behavior—*finally unlock your parenting potential.* Use this handbook to move beyond typical discipline techniques and begin creating an environment based on mutual respect, emotional safety, and positive, open communication. *Respectful Parents, Respectful Kids* offers *7 Simple Keys* to discover the mutual respect and nurturing relationships you've been looking for.

Use these 7 Keys to:

- Set firm limits without using demands or coercion
- Achieve mutual respect without being submissive
- Successfully prevent, reduce, and resolve conflicts
- Empower your kids to open up, co-operate, and realize their full potential
- Make your home a *No-Fault Zone* where trust thrives

With a combined 45 years of parent education and teaching experience, the authors offer you a refreshing alternative. Activities, stories, and resources will help you immediately apply these seven keys to even your toughest parenting situations.

Learn Powerful, Practical Skills to:

- Successfully handle disagreements or problem behaviors
- Express yourself so you're heard and respected
- Transform anger and conflict into co-operation and trust
- Motivate your kids to willingly contribute
- Create outstanding lifelong relationships with your kids

"This delightful book shows parents how to get the best results for their kids with respectful tools that are neither punitive nor permissive."
> **—Jane Nelsen**, coauthor, *The Positive Discipline series*

"This is the best parent read since *How To Talk So Kids Will Listen!*"
> **—Brenda Harari, Ph.D.**, HEART in Education

Available from PuddleDancer Press, the Center for Nonviolent Communication, all major bookstores, and Amazon.com. Distributed by Independent Publisher's Group: 800-888-4741.

SAVE 10% at NonviolentCommunication.com with coupon code: **bookads**

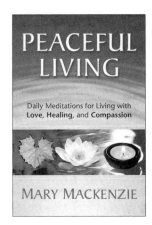

Peaceful Living

Daily Meditations for Living With Love, Healing, and Compassion

by Mary Mackenzie

$19.95 — Trade Paper 5x7.5, 448pp
ISBN: 978-1-892005-19-9

Live More Authentically and Peacefully Than You Ever Dreamed Possible

In this gathering of wisdom, Mary Mackenzie empowers you to change the course of your life for the better. With each of the 366 daily meditations you will learn new ways of viewing familiar, everyday situations and discover tools to transform those situations into opportunities for connection and personal growth.

Peaceful Living goes beyond daily affirmations, providing the skills and consciousness you need to transform relationships, heal pain, and discover the life-enriching meaning behind even the most trying situations. Begin each day centered and connected to yourself and your values. Direct the course of your life toward your deepest hopes and needs. Ground yourself in the power of compassionate, conscious living.

Discover the life-enriching benefits of *Peaceful Living:*

- Create an empowered, purposeful life free of fear, shame, or guilt

- Deepen your emotional connections with your partner, colleagues, family, and friends

- Hear the needs behind whatever anyone does or says

- Transform judgment and criticism into understanding and connection

Available from PuddleDancer Press, the Center for Nonviolent Communication, all major bookstores, and Amazon.com. Distributed by Independent Publisher's Group: 800-888-4741.

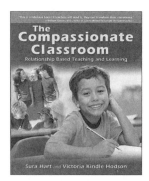

The Compassionate Classroom

Relationship Based Teaching and Learning

by Sura Hart and Victoria Kindle Hodson

$17.95 – Trade Paper 7.5x9.25, 208pp
ISBN: 978-1-892005-06-9

When Compassion Thrives, So Does Learning.

The Compassionate Classroom is a long awaited how-to guide for educators who care about the creating a safe, productive learning environment. With 45 years combined teaching experience, Sura Hart and Victoria Kindle Hodson merge recent discoveries in brain research with the proven skills of Nonviolent Communication and come to a bold conclusion—when compassion thrives, so does learning.

Learn powerful skills to create an emotionally safe learning environment where academic excellence thrives. Build trust, reduce conflict, improve co-operation, and maximize the potential of each student as you create relationship-centered classrooms. This how-to guide is perfect for any educator, homeschool parent, administrator, or mentor. Customizable exercises, activities, charts, and cutouts make it easy for educators to create lesson plans for a day, a week, or an entire school year.

"Education is not simply about teachers covering a curriculum; it is a dance of relationships. *The Compassionate Classroom* presents both the case for teaching compassionately and a wide range of practical things to do and say with children that will help to create and sustain a culture of meaningful intellectual work."

—Tim Seldin, president, Montessori Foundation

"Today's teachers can create a Planet of Peace. The communication process you will learn by reading this book is the cornerstone."

—Robert Muller, former Assistant Secretary General of the United Nations and co-founder of the University for Peace in Costa Rica

"This is a fabulous book! If teachers will read it, they can transform their classrooms."

—William Glasser, M.D., author of *Schools Without Failure* and *The Quality School*

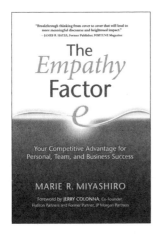

The Empathy Factor

Your Competitive Advantage for Personal, Team, and Business Success

by Marie R. Miyashiro, A.P.R.

$19.95 — Trade Paper 6x9, 256pp
ISBN: 978-1-892005-25-0

"Breakthrough thinking from cover to cover. *The Empathy Factor* will help thoughtful business people add substance and dimension to relationships within the workforce—colleagues and customers."

—JAMES B. HAYES, Former Publisher, FORTUNE Magazine

In this groundbreaking book, award-winning communication and organizational strategist Marie Miyashiro explores the missing element leaders must employ to build profits and productivity in the new economy—Empathy.

Building from the latest research about organizational effectiveness, emotional aptitude in the workplace, and brain science, Miyashiro offers both real-world insight and a practical framework to bring the transformative power of empathy to your entire organization.

Miyashiro's approach combines more than 26 years of experience advising for-profit companies, government agencies, and nonprofits to substantially improve their organizational communication with a proven, world-renowned process from the largest empathy-based community in the world.

The Empathy Factor takes Dr. Marshall Rosenberg's work developing Compassionate Communication into the business community by introducing *Integrated Clarity®*—a powerful framework you can use to understand and effectively meet the critical needs of your organization without compromising those of your employees or customers.

Available from PuddleDancer Press, the Center for Nonviolent Communication, all major bookstores, and Amazon.com. Distributed by Independent Publisher's Group: 800-888-4741.

SAVE 10% at NonviolentCommunication.com with coupon code: **bookads**

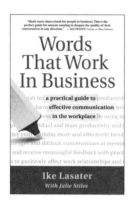

Words That Work In Business

A Practical Guide to Effective Communication in the Workplace

by Ike Lasater
with Julie Stiles

$12.95 — Trade Paper 5-3/8x8-3/8, 144pp
ISBN: 978-1-892005-01-4

Do You Want to Be Happier, More Effective, and Experience Less Stress at Work?

Do you wish for more respectful work relationships? To move beyond gossip and power struggles, to improved trust and productivity? If you've ever wondered if just one person can positively affect work relationships and company culture, regardless of your position, this book offers a resounding "yes." The key is shifting how we think and talk.

Former attorney-turned-mediator, Ike Lasater, offers practical communication skills matched with recognizable work scenarios to help anyone address the most common workplace relationship challenges. Learn proven communication skills to: Enjoy your workday more; effectively handle difficult conversations; reduce workplace conflict and stress; improve individual and team productivity; be more effective at meetings; and give and receive meaningful feedback.

Save an additional 10% at NonviolentCommunication.com with coupon code: **bookads**

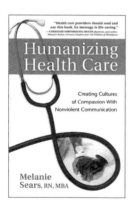

Humanizing Health Care

Creating Cultures of Compassion With Nonviolent Communication

By Melanie Sears, RN, MBA

$9.95 — Trade Paper 5-3/8x8-3/8, 112pp
ISBN: 978-1-892005-26-7

It's Time to Address the *Real* Crisis in Health Care

Now that U.S. policymakers have tackled the first major health care policy reform in history, it's also time to take a candid look at the dysfunctional culture that has such a dire effect on the quality of patient care. In this engaging book, Melanie Sears, RN, MBA, leverages more than 25 years of nursing experience to do just that. From domination-style management, fear- and judgment-based practitioner relationships, and a poignant separation between physical, mental, and emotional care, the costs of these factors is enormous. Sears argues that the most effective way to evolve this problematic culture is to shift the language used by those providing care.

Available from PuddleDancer Press, the Center for Nonviolent Communication, all major bookstores, and Amazon.com. Distributed by Independent Publisher's Group: 800-888-4741.

Being Me, Loving You: *A Practical Guide to Extraordinary Relationships* **by Marshall B. Rosenberg, Ph.D.** • Watch your relationships strengthen as you learn to think of love as something you "do," something you give freely from the heart. 80pp • **$8.95**

Getting Past the Pain Between Us: *Healing and Reconciliation Without Compromise* **by Marshall B. Rosenberg, Ph.D.** • Learn simple steps to create the heartfelt presence necessary for lasting healing to occur—great for mediators, counselors, families, and couples. 48pp • **$8.95**

Graduating From Guilt: *Six Steps to Overcome Guilt and Reclaim Your Life* **by Holly Michelle Eckert** • The burden of guilt leaves us stuck, stressed, and feeling like we can never measure up. Through a proven six-step process, this book helps liberate you from the toxic guilt, blame, and shame you carry. 96pp • **$9.95**

Humanizing Health Care: *Creating Cultures of Compassion With Nonviolent Communication* **by Melanie Sears, RN, MBA** • Leveraging more than 25 years nursing experience, Melanie demonstrates the profound effectiveness of NVC to create lasting, positive improvements to patient care and the health care workplace. 112pp • **$9.95**

Parenting From Your Heart: *Sharing the Gifts of Compassion, Connection, and Choice* **by Inbal Kashtan** • Filled with insight and practical skills, this booklet will help you transform your parenting to address every day challenges. 48pp • **$8.95**

Raising Children Compassionately: *Parenting the Nonviolent Communication Way* **by Marshall B. Rosenberg, Ph.D.** • Learn to create a mutually respectful, enriching family dynamic filled with heartfelt communication. 32pp • **$7.95**

The Surprising Purpose of Anger: *Beyond Anger Management: Finding the Gift* **by Marshall B. Rosenberg, Ph.D.** • Marshall shows you how to use anger to discover what you need, and then how to meet your needs in more constructive, healthy ways. 48pp • **$8.95**

Teaching Children Compassionately: *How Students and Teachers Can Succeed With Mutual Understanding* **by Marshall B. Rosenberg, Ph.D.** • In this national keynote address to Montessori educators, Marshall describes his progressive, radical approach to teaching that centers on compassionate connection. 48pp • **$8.95**

We Can Work It Out: *Resolving Conflicts Peacefully and Powerfully* **by Marshall B. Rosenberg, Ph.D.** • Practical suggestions for fostering empathic connection, genuine co-operation, and satisfying resolutions in even the most difficult situations. 32pp • **$7.95**

What's Making You Angry? *10 Steps to Transforming Anger So Everyone Wins* **by Shari Klein and Neill Gibson** • A powerful, step-by-step approach to transform anger to find healthy, mutually satisfying outcomes. 32pp • **$7.95**

Available from www.NonviolentCommunication.com, www.CNVC.org, Amazon.com and all bookstores. Distributed by IPG: 800-888-4741

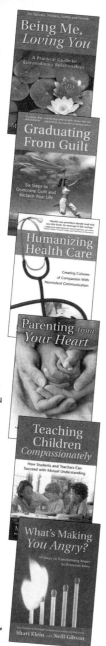

SAVE 10% at NonviolentCommunication.com with coupon code: **bookads**

About the Author

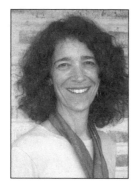

Sylvia Haskvitz, registered dietitian (since 1983) and CNVC Certified Trainer with the Center for Nonviolent (since 1989), played with both of her lifelong passions in writing this book—food/food psychology and Compassionate Communication. Sylvia has been sharing NVC in a variety of venues for twenty-two years. She is the past host of the radio show, "Call in a Conflict," the former television host for "People Skills," and her essay, "Enemy Images" was published in the book, *Healing Our Planet, Healing Ourselves*. Sylvia offers communication coaching, consulting, and facilitation to individuals, groups, and organizations by phone and in person throughout the world. She lives in Tucson, Arizona, and her website is eatbychoice.net.